routine ey

WW 141 HAR £24·99

For Elsevier Butterworth-Heinemann:

Publishing Director: Caroline Makepeace
Commissioning Editor: Robert Edwards
Development Editor: Kim Benson
Project Manager: Anne Dickie
Design Direction: George Ajayi

eye essentials

routine eye examination

William Harvey MCOptom
Visiting Clinician and Director of Visual Impairment Clinic,
City University, London, UK
Professional Programme Tutor for Boots Opticians Ltd
Clinical Editor, Optician, Reed Business Information, Sutton, UK

Andrew Franklin FBCO D.Orth DCLP
Professional Programme Tutor, Boots Opticians Examiner,
College of Optometrists
Optometrist in private practice, Gloucestershire, UK

SERIES EDITORS
Sandip Doshi PhD, MCOptom
Optometrist in private practice, Hove, East Sussex, UK
Examiner, College of Optometrists, London, UK
Formerly Clinical Editor, Optician

William Harvey MCOptom
Visiting Clinician and Director of Visual Impairment Clinic, City University, London, UK
Professional Programme Tutor for Boots Opticians Ltd
Clinical Editor, Optician, Reed Business Information, Sutton, UK

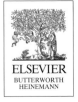

ELSEVIER
BUTTERWORTH
HEINEMANN

EDINBURGH LONDON NEW YORK OXFORD
PHILADELPHIA ST LOUIS SYDNEY TORONTO 2005

ELSEVIER
BUTTERWORTH
HEINEMANN

© 2005, Elsevier Limited. All rights reserved.
First published 2005

No part of this publication may be reproduced, stored in a retrieval system, or transmitted in any form or by any means, electronic, mechanical, photocopying, recording or otherwise, without either the prior permission of the publishers or a licence permitting restricted copying in the United Kingdom issued by the Copyright Licensing Agency, 90 Tottenham Court Road, London W1T 4LP. Permissions may be sought directly from Elsevier's Health Sciences Rights Department in Philadelphia, USA: (+1) 215 238 7869, fax: (+1) 215 238 2239, e-mail: healthpermissions@elsevier.com. You may also complete your request on-line via the Elsevier homepage (http://www.elsevier.com), by selecting 'Customer Support' and then 'Obtaining Permissions'.

ISBN 0 7506 8852 1

British Library Cataloguing in Publication Data
A catalogue record for this book is available from the British Library.

Library of Congress Cataloging in Publication Data
A catalog record for this book is available from the Library of Congress.

Note
Knowledge and best practice in this field are constantly changing. As new research and experience broaden our knowledge, changes in practice, treatment and drug therapy may become necessary or appropriate. Readers are advised to check the most current information provided (i) on procedures featured or (ii) by the manufacturer of each product to be administered, to verify the recommended dose or formula, the method and duration of administration, and contraindications. It is the responsibility of the practitioner, relying on their own experience and knowledge of the patient, to make diagnoses, to determine dosages and the best treatment for each individual patient, and to take all appropriate safety precautions. To the fullest extent of the law, neither the publisher nor the editors assumes any liability for any injury and/or damage to persons or property arising from this publication.

ELSEVIER   your source for books,
journals and multimedia
in the health sciences

www.elsevierhealth.com

The
publisher's
policy is to use
paper manufactured
from sustainable forests

Printed in China

Contents

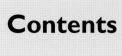
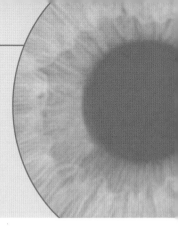

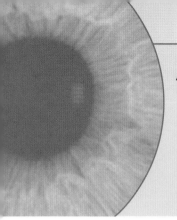

Acknowledgments

Thanks to Heidi, Tallulah, Kitty, Spike and Napalm Death

Bill Harvey

Thanks to Ngaire, Joe, Lili and also Rocco the Hamster whose sterling work on the wheel inspired me to ever greater efforts (he's dead now!)

Andy Franklin

Foreword

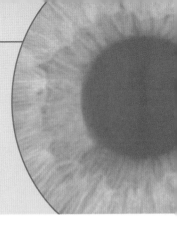

Eye Essentials is a series of books intended to cover the core skills required by the eye care practitioner in general and/or specialised practice. It consists of books covering a wide range of topics ranging from: routine eye examination to assessment and management of low vision; assessment and investigative techniques to digital imaging; case reports and law to contact lenses.

Authors known for their interest and expertise in their particular subject have contributed books to this series. The reader will know many of them as they have published widely within their respective fields. Each author has addressed key topics in their subject in a practical rather than theoretical approach hence each book has a particular relevance to everyday practice.

Each book follows a similar format and has been designed to enable the reader to ascertain information easily and quickly. Each chapter has been produced in a user-friendly format, thus providing the reader with a rapid-reference book that is easy to use in the consulting room or in the practitioner's free time.

Optometry and dispensing optics are continually developing professions with the emphasis in each being redefined as we learn more from research and as technology stamps its mark. The *Eye Essentials* series is particularly relevant to the practitioner's requirements and as such will appeal to students,

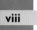

graduates sitting professional examinations and qualified practitioners alike. We hope you enjoy reading these books as much as we have enjoyed producing them.

Sandip Doshi
Bill Harvey

1
Introduction

For the majority of optometrists, routine eye examination is the activity that occupies most of their professional life. The working day may be punctuated by contact lens appointments, dispensing or management, but "The Routine" is there like a heartbeat. It becomes an extension of the practitioner, and will eventually become as personal as a fingerprint. This is a desirable evolution, driven by the acquisition of knowledge and experience, but it does create problems for those starting out. The diversity of methods and interpretations encountered, even in undergraduate clinics, tends to create confusion rather than the wide breadth of useful variation intended. This is perhaps a controversial statement, but it is based on experience.

The term "routine examination" becomes most familiar to optometrists as part of their professional qualifying examinations. The term is used to describe the various procedures required during a full eye examination in order to properly assess both the optical status of a patient (and be able to prescribe an appropriate optical correction) and the ocular health.

For the best part of a decade, the authors have been members of a team that was created to help optometric graduates through their pre-registration year and professional qualifying examinations (PQE). The job involved regular teaching in undergraduate clinics, as well as on postgraduate courses in preparation for the PQE. Experience as examiners for the College of Optometrists was also brought to bear, so over the years we have seen a lot of people go through university clinics, pre-registration year and their professional examinations.

Initially, "Routine" gave us more headaches than any other section of the PQE and had traditionally the poorest first-time pass rate of any of the sections. We tried the usual refresher course approach, but it seemed to have no effect on the pass rate, though it did in other sections. It was only when we became more proactive that the results started to improve measurably. Essentially we caught the pre-regs early in their year with a routine designed by a number of examiners, in an attempt to avoid some of the confusion that we were seeing in our tutees. The process involved one of us writing out an instruction manual which was then reviewed by a further ten examiners, who were between them teaching in all of the optometry departments then in existence. To everyone's surprise we managed to settle all disputes without war breaking out. In fact, there really wasn't that much that was controversial at all. The final version was then agreed and the result passed on to the graduate optometrists as they began their pre-registration year. It is from this work that much of this book has been developed, though it is hoped that it will prove as useful to a pre-registration optometrist as it may be to an experienced practitioner who, through years of developing a particular routine, may wish to revise a lesser used technique.

Those entering the profession from university often have little reliable basis upon which to make informed choices, due to lack of contact with patients during their undergraduate period. Choices between different techniques during an eye examination become randomized, likely to be influenced more by ease of application or under the influence of one particular supervisor. What new practitioners need, we believe, is for experienced practitioners to take the responsibility of choosing a method that works, rather than a range that might or might not. As the new practitioner gains experience, they can begin to evolve their own routine, provided the roots are sound. The methods described are not the only ones, and maybe not even the best ones, but they have been thoroughly road-tested, both in the professional examinations and in practice. The authors have between them worked in every type of optometric practice from high street to hospital, and from locum to LASIK clinic, and these are the methods we have used. The book may prove particularly useful to those approaching the newly trialed pre-registration year, with its assessor visits and final examinations.

The working environment is composed of legal, moral and commercial elements. Guidance on what constitutes a proper examination has been provided by the College of Optometrists Code of Ethics and Guidance for Professional Conduct, which the General Optical Council tends to regard as the "peer view" in disciplinary cases. On the routine eye examination the guideline is as follows:

> "The optometrist has a duty to carry out whatever tests are necessary to determine the patient's needs for vision care as to both sight and health. The exact format and content will be determined by both the practitioner's professional judgment and the minimum legal requirements".

The legal requirements are defined in the Sight Testing (Examination and Prescription) (Number 2) Regulations issued in 1998, following measures contained in the Health and Medicines Act 1989. The relevant sentences are these:

> "(1) When a doctor or optician tests the sight of another person it shall be his duty
>   (a) to perform for the purpose of detecting sign of injury, disease or abnormality in the eye or elsewhere
>   (i) an examination of the external surface of the eye and its immediate vicinity
>   (ii) an intraocular examination, either by means of an ophthalmoscope or by such other means as the doctor or optician considers appropriate
>   (iii) such additional examinations as appear to the doctor or optician to be clinically necessary".

The essential message here is that if you test someone's eyes with the aim of issuing a visual correction, you can't just do a refraction. You have to screen the health of their eyes as well. This fact has shaped the structure of the routine as well as making its internal logic rather more difficult to follow at first. There are two end points rather than one and the efficient organization of the routine requires that both end points are arrived at with the minimum expenditure of effort and in a reasonable time.

What constitutes a reasonable time is open to debate. At undergraduate level, examinations are measured by the calendar rather than the clock, yet essentially the same ground is covered in 20 minutes in what is often rather disparagingly called "High Street practice". Purists may sniff, yet the 20-minute sight test interval, which is the de facto industry standard, has not apparently caused widespread loss of sight among the population, and the remake rate has not gone into orbit. So it seems likely to stay. In many smaller practices, 30 minutes is allowed between appointments, but that often includes 10 minutes for dispensing. In larger practices, with dispensing a separate function, tonometry, fields and the use of autorefractors are often delegated to support staff. Provided that these staff are well trained, this can save considerable time. Either way, as a fully-fledged optometrist you may well have about 20 minutes maximum to carry out a "routine".

The other factor that needs to be taken into account is the patient. Research has indicated that they are unimpressed by prolonged sight testing. In fact, as will be discussed in Chapter 2, if the quality of the communication and the technique is good enough, the actual testing time bears little influence upon the patient's satisfaction with their assessment, their recall of information, and their compliance with any instructions given.

The routine can be regarded as a process of information gathering and decision-making and the fundamental difference between the undergraduate refraction and that performed by the fully-fledged practitioner is the approach to the gathering of information.

Undergraduate refractions adopt what has been called a "database" approach. The less polite term for this is "box-filling". Essentially, the same information is collected for every patient, whether it is directly relevant or not. The advantage of this approach in university clinics is that it is less likely that any essential information is missed or not recorded, so the supervisor will have enough information to make the clinical decision at the end of the clinic. Unfortunately, a drawback to this approach is that, for the student, information gathering and recording becomes an end in itself, and the crucial process of clinical decision-making becomes a delegated function. Furthermore, much of the information gathered will be essentially useless, which wastes time. If this approach was used extensively by experienced practitioners, the number of patients seen in a working day would be uneconomic and arguably less effective clinically.

The experienced practitioner tends to have a smaller database to fill, though a certain amount of information is required for legal reasons, and some baseline information is useful to compare against future values (e.g. intraocular pressures, visual fields) for the early detection of trends. What was once "routine" may have become "subroutine", brought in when the patient's symptoms and history, or clinical findings, indicate their relevance. The more knowledge and experience the practitioner accumulates, the better this approach works. It follows that the routine is not fixed, it evolves. Not so many years ago, optometrists ascribed enormous significance to small differences in intraocular pressures and to the presence or absence of visual field changes, while largely ignoring the optic disc. Now we know that half of all glaucomas are normotensive, and that a patient can lose half of their nerve fiber layer without displaying a glaucomatous field loss, our approach to early glaucoma has changed significantly.

It seems that optometrists will shortly be involved in the prescribing of therapeutic agents to treat a range of anterior eye conditions. The type of consultation needed to do this well is unlikely to be the same as one resulting in a pair of bifocals. For the moment, we shall concentrate on the more usual type of consultation, where the object is to arrive at a suitable optical correction, if required, and to screen the health of the eyes and adnexa. The precise order of the tests used will vary from practitioner to practitioner, and in many cases it makes little difference. However, there are some general principles to apply.

Tests with the patient wearing their accustomed correction should be done before testing without it, in order to get an idea of their normal status before the testing process completely disrupts it. Tests should be done in such an order that each test makes subsequent ones easier. If you want to know what target to use for your cover test, it is helpful to know what the patient's visual acuity is. If you are about to start retinoscopy, knowledge of the symptoms and history and aided and unaided vision will help you to make a sensible choice of correcting lens, thus saving time. At the very least, they should not make the next test more difficult, or invalid. An example here would be to perform a fixation disparity test after a dissociation test (though this is frequently done), or to cover one up during the test and say "which line can you see now?" Binocular tests should precede ones that dissociate unless the reverse is unavoidable, and binocular vision should be stabilized before it is tested. Similarly, a patient with maculopathy should not be examined with an ophthalmoscope before all measurements of vision are completed, as the resultant after-image may take some time to clear. In most other cases, ophthalmoscopy can be done before or after the refraction. If done before, any pathological findings can be taken into account when you come to refract. Leaving ophthalmoscopy to the end allows refractive findings to point toward likely pathology, prevents a disabling after image, and allows the patient time to get used to the practitioner before the necessary invasion of personal space that accompanies ophthalmoscopy. But most of the time either way works just as well.

Table 1.1 shows a suggested order for a routine examination of the type that tends to be performed in professional examinations and assessor's visits, applying the principles discussed above. But it is just a suggestion.

Table 1.1 **Suggested order of routine eye examination and chapter reference for each procedure**

Order	Procedure	Chapter
1	Patient personal details	2
2	Focimetry (if applicable)	
3	History and symptoms	2
4	Corrected vision distance binocular/right/left	3
5	Cover test with Rx distance (if applicable)*	4
6	Corrected vision near binocular/right/left	3
7	Cover test with Rx near (if applicable)*	4
8	Unaided vision distance binocular/right/left	3
9	Cover test without Rx distance (if applicable)*	4
10	Unaided vision near binocular/right/left	3
11	Cover test without Rx near (if applicable)*	4
12	Near point of convergence	4

(Continued)

Table 1.1 **Suggested order of routine eye examination and chapter reference for each procedure—Cont'd**

Order	Procedure	Chapter
13	Motility	4
14	Pupils (direct, consensual, near, afferent)	5
15	Confrontation/perimetry	6
16	External eye/ophthalmoscopy[†]	10
17	Measure PD and adjust trial frame	7
18	Retinoscopy	7
19	Best vision sphere	8
20	Cross-cylinder	8
21	Fixation disparity for distance with Rx	4
22	Cover test for distance with Rx	4
23	Amplitude of accommodation	9
24	Adjust trial frame for near (if applicable)	9
25	Reading addition	9
26	Stereopsis (if indicated)	4
27	Fixation disparity for near with Rx	4
28	Cover test for near with Rx	4
29	External eye/ophthalmoscopy[†]	10
30	Prescribing and advice	11

*If the patient's symptoms suggest a binocular problem, it may be worth doing fixation disparity with their own correction before the cover test.
[†]These are optional positions in most cases, but for patients with maculopathy it is advisable to avoid glare until all acuity measurements are completed.

2
History and symptoms

Significance of history and symptoms

It is a safe assumption that a patient will attend for an eye examination for a reason. This reason may range from simple response to a posted reminder from a practice to the reporting of a specific visual or ocular symptom. It is often stated that the first question an optometrist might ask is "Why are you here?" If the reason for attendance is not addressed then it cannot be deemed a successful examination. If the reason for attendance is to be investigated properly, then the optometrist must ask pertinent questions to place the patient requirement in its appropriate context. This process of gathering information which will be discussed in this chapter.

A thorough initial interview with a patient has the following advantages:

- Baseline data may be recorded which aids accuracy and efficiency in future examinations of a patient. It allows for monitoring of any changes over time and provides clues as to the success or relevance of any previous interventions.
- Careful questioning allows the optometrist to discover the nature of any problem relating to a patient's vision or ocular health.
- It allows a good rapport between the optometrist and the patient to be established.
- Allied information may be gained that may allow the optometrist to offer advice beyond the presenting needs of the patient. For example, if it is discovered that a patient with glaucoma has a middle-aged brother, or that a high myope has had a child recently, the practitioner may be able to offer practical eyecare advice.
- The information gained at the beginning of the examination allows the optometrist to adapt the clinical assessment to meet the needs of the patient. Often the decision to omit certain tests as irrelevant is based upon information gained from the patient, for example not measuring amplitude of accommodation in a patient once they have disclosed their age.

The information may also impact on the use of further investigations; for example, a patient with asthenopic symptoms with a cover test result showing a poorly controlled phoria may warrant further investigation of fusional reserves or fixation disparity.

The adaptation of the clinical procedures to meet the requirements of the patient has been described as a problem-oriented examination as opposed to a checklist examination where a set pattern of techniques are applied to every patient. It may be argued that basing the design of the examination to meet the needs of a patient as gleaned from a thorough initial interview allows the optometrist to use their time more efficiently and to reach an accurate conclusion without the need for carrying out unnecessary tests. On the other hand, this must be tempered by the practitioner's skill in inferring when the patient has given adequate or accurate information. As will become clear from the forthcoming case examples, one may not always be given the full, or even the true picture by the patient. Furthermore, there are many examples where a condition may be detected in a patient with no predisposing symptoms or history, such as open-angle glaucoma. Therefore, an approach based purely on the presenting problem may overshadow this consideration.

- The recording of accurate data based upon a history and symptoms may have legal implications in that, if a problem occurs subsequent to an examination, then clear recorded evidence that the optometrist asked questions relating to a condition at the time of the examination is important. Asking about systemic medications with a patient who subsequently suffered an adverse ocular reaction, or about the nature of perceived flashing lights in a high myope who developed a retinal detachment some years later, may prove crucial in any subsequent litigation.

The role of auxiliary staff

It is important to remember that in a great many cases, the initial information gathering may be carried out by a receptionist or trained optical or clinical assistant. The use of such staff has proved popular in the operation of many of the usually automated procedures that provide useful baseline data to the optometrist, for example tonometry, fields, focimetry and autorefraction. The argument for this approach has been that the optometrist may then interpret the information gained and use their time more effectively in following up this data.

Similarly, a clinical assistant may record patient details relating to age, address, date of last eye examination and so on. Arguments for this approach, again, center upon the more efficient use of professional time. There has therefore been an argument for expanding this information-gathering role to include assistants asking questions commonly considered to be part of the traditional history and symptoms, so allowing the optometrist more time to investigate the patient which would otherwise have been spent asking questions. Such questions might include asking about the reason for the patient's visit, family history, medication and so on. However, arguments for limiting this role include:

- The initial questioning by the optometrist establishes a rapport which facilitates subsequent flow of information.
- A skilled optometrist may usefully use probing questions based upon responses to initial questions.
- The patient may feel less of a bond of trust or confidentiality if imparting clinical information to more than one person and so limit their responses accordingly.

In our experience, a good working relationship with a trained optical or clinical assistant may save valuable time that may be spent more usefully in a more detailed assessment.

The nature of the information

The information obtained during the initial part of the consultation is usually concerned with previous events in a patient's life concerning their optical, ocular or general health state and any significant recent or presenting symptoms or known signs of concern. The gathering of information occurs at two levels:

1. **Cognitive.** This concerns the acquisition of (known) facts and details regarding, for example, any blurred vision, pain, or health problems. Much of the literature regarding useful questioning techniques and patient handling is often concerned with the cognitive information.

2. **Affective.** This concerns the appraisal of overall "feeling" about a patient that is gained during an interaction and is often driven by nonverbal aspects. It is possible to have two consultations based around two similar problems, such as a particular ametropia, but the two patients giving very different signals to the practitioner may heavily influence the outcome. If a patient is very anxious or has very precise demands, the practitioner may perceive this even if the actual questions and answers follow an identical pattern in each case. The skill of the practitioner in detecting and interpreting such subtle nuances is very difficult to teach and is something that most gain with experience throughout their professional life. Even in a problem-oriented approach, nonverbal cues may help the practitioner to gain an insight into the underlying problem. A subconscious appraisal of a patient's personality may, for example, lead one to quiz a patient further about a headache which the patient may be dismissing offhand as an irrelevant feature.

The ideal situation for overall patient appraisal is therefore a balance of both cognitive and affective appraisal of the patient and this process continues from the outset to the conclusion of the consultation. It may also influence further interactions between the practitioner and the same patient in future consultations and forms the basis of establishing a good patient rapport. Most practitioners have found that subsequent consultations are facilitated if previous ones have been effective.

In gaining affective information, an optometrist skilled in picking up nonverbal cues may be able to reach a more accurate conclusion for their patient and so a brief reminder of nonverbal behavior would seem useful.

Interpreting nonverbal information: gaining affective information

Before a word has been uttered, an optometrist may already be gaining useful information regarding a patient. On a specific note, an unusual head posture may indicate an extra ocular muscle problem, an unsteady gait, a significant field loss or a vestibulocochlear problem. On a more general note, and one that applies to all clinical situations, the nonverbal behavior of a patient gives useful affective information and may allow some judgment of the patient's personality, state of mind or even general health.

In making affective judgments it is always worth remembering the dangers of stereotyping. Judging a patient totally on nonverbal behavior, particularly appearance, is fraught with danger. The assumptions that the frail pensioner responds best to gentle questioning, that the tattooed muscle-bound night-club bouncer prefers colloquial chat or, worse still, that a child needs to be talked to in the most simplistic of manners are all clearly risky. Stereotyping, in as much as it is a function of our own experience-based learning process, is difficult to avoid but in the context of information gathering, every effort should be made to control our own natural prejudices.

There now follows a list of nonverbal cues and some notes as to their interpretation.

Body contact

A handshake on first meeting the patient may be interpreted as warm and friendly, but equally may be considered as intrusive and unsettling. When a patient is not known, it is a risky procedure.

Proximity

A patient who stands very close to the optometrist on initial meeting may be of an aggressive nature, or this may be a sign of insecurity on the patient's part. The distance between two people gives strong nonverbal messages, dependent to some extent on cultural factors and experience, and so also should be borne in mind by the practitioner when sitting down to begin the examination.

Orientation

The position of an individual relative to another gives some indication of the interrelationship independent of their proximity. A person positioned higher up than another is usually perceived as being in a dominant position, possibly a legacy of the relationship between parents and children. For this reason it is preferable for the optometrist to be at the same vertical level as a patient to maintain equality in the relationship, so facilitating the flow of information. When shown silent films of professionals or managers greeting patients or clients and welcoming them into their consulting rooms, most viewers taking part in one experiment accurately established which were the more friendly. The professional who moved toward the patient at initial meeting tended to be rated as more friendly, the one who waited for the patient to approach less friendly but thought to be more senior or of higher rank. In a situation where a patient has a specific and potentially serious problem about which they are worried, a more formal approach may be appropriate. In general, surveys have indicated that, for routine eye examinations, patients prefer a friendly environment. In examining children, a more formal approach is usually best avoided.

Body language

The way we control our body movements during interaction is very important in dictating the nature of the communication. The complexity of body language has meant that it is usually studied as comprising many individual components (or "kinesics"). These include the following:

Body posture
Body posture may signal an individual's emotional state, such as anxious or nervous, or the attitude to other

individuals, such as arrogance or extroversion. Standing erect with the head tilted back and hands on the hips may indicate the desire to dominate or an assumed stance of authority. Conversely, head bowed and shoulders hunched forward are often signs of submission or insecurity. Cultural influences and fashions are important in interpretation of body postures. Similarly, the background of an individual, such as previous military training, may have an effect on behavior.

Though nervousness is difficult to manipulate, body posture is easier to voluntarily change and it is important for the optometrist

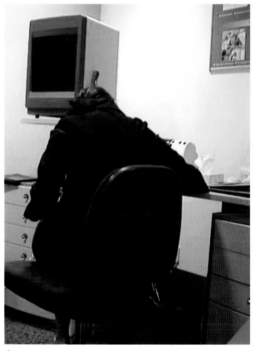

A

Figure 2.1 *(A)* Poor positioning for information gathering *(Continued)*

to appear relaxed and at ease during an examination. Outward display of nervousness or anxiety can hinder the flow of information between practitioner and patient.

Body posture may be interpreted as showing how well the practitioner is listening. It is generally recommended that the practitioner face the patient directly such that the axis of the patient's shoulders is parallel to that of the practitioner. This is referred to, rather obviously, as facing the patient squarely and may be facilitated by use of a clipboard for carrying the record card to avoid continually turning away to make notes. A forward lean may also enhance the appearance of attentiveness by the practitioner (Figure 2.1).

Gestures
Movements of the hands, feet or other parts of the body may be used to communicate definite messages. Gestures are very closely

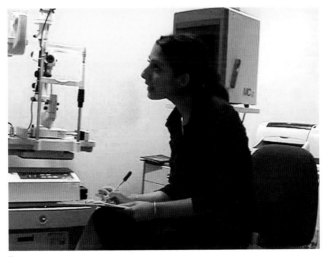

B

Figure 2.1 *(B)* Leaning forward, maintaining good eye contact.

associated with speech and are often essential to communicate the full intended message.

Head-nods

By acknowledging receipt and understanding of information, a head-nod acts as a powerful "reinforcer", a reward or encouragement to a speaker to continue. An occasional nod encourages the other individual to continue speaking while a rapid succession of nods may indicate that the "nodder" wishes to interject.

Facial expression

The patient will tend to look directly at the practitioner's face during communication and hence the expression is a powerful social cue. Unlike most animals that use facial expression as a major form of communication, the ability of humans to control expression irrespective of the emotion "behind the façade" reduces its impact. It does, however, increase its usefulness in the clinical environment, for example in disguising nerves on the part of the practitioner, or hiding some concern about the patient's ocular or general well-being.

Eyes

The influence of the eyes in communicating is quite out of proportion to the physical effort needed for their control. Other individuals may detect the dilation of the pupils under the action of the sympathetic nervous system during states of heightened emotional activity. The clinical value of this phenomenon may be mostly confined to the subtle, possibly subconscious, appraisal of the other individual's emotional state.

The speaker will use eye contact to help convey the information, interruptions of gaze helping to reinforce speech, and to monitor the state of awareness of the listener. The listener will give information about attentiveness and help to regulate the pattern of speech by eye contact. Individuals will maintain eye contact nearly twice as long when listening as when speaking. The listener usually maintains longer glances and the away-glances are shorter. Practitioners who avoid eye contact may be perceived as uninterested or inattentive or shy. The importance

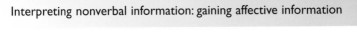
of the optometrist appearing to be a good listener cannot be over-emphasized. Making eye contact in the very early stage of a consultation is a powerful aid to establishing rapport. Direct and steady eye contact makes a speaker appear confident and steadfast, so evoking professional authority without appearing dominant or aggressive. This may be important in reassuring an uncertain patient or in giving information that could be distressing to the patient, for example during the explanation of the need for referral.

Appearance

It is widely accepted that the healthcare professional should appear neat and respectable. This is what patients expect, and so enhances the initial orientation of the patient to allow rapport to be established. It may also communicate a "caring" attitude to the patient, establishing a confidence in the practitioner's own standards of self-hygiene and personal care. Occasionally, changes in appearance may give important clinical information to a practitioner. Deterioration in a patient's appearance over successive appointments may indicate problems with their coping generally, for example a patient with visual impairment who has started to become depressed and resigned.

Nonverbal speech patterns: paralinguistics

The same words may be spoken in different ways and within a different context to communicate completely different messages. The various ways of enhancing the spoken words are called paralanguage or paralinguistics and they include:

Intonation

Changing the emphasis of component words may change the overall meaning. Take for instance the following statement:
"My general health is reasonably good."

- Emphasis of "**reasonably**" leads one to infer that health is not "totally good".
- Emphasis of "**is**" suggests a disagreement with a view held by someone else that the health may not be quite as good as originally thought.

- Emphasis of "**general**" may indicate that there may be a problem considered minor by the speaker and so not worthy of being described as a general health problem, such as a watery eye.
- Emphasis of "**my**" may indicate a wish to tell of a health problem experienced by someone else.

In fact this simple six-word statement could have many implications. Appropriate use and interpretation of emphasis and intonation by a practitioner is an effective way of communicating and receiving information.

Rate of speech

Speaking very quickly may not only confuse a patient, but may convey nerves or anxiety on the part of the speaker. Speaking inappropriately slowly may leave a patient considering the practitioner to be uninterested or even patronizing. The rate of speech of the practitioner may be adjusted after an assessment of the ability of the patient to process information. If there is a language difficulty or a hearing deficit then a slower rate of speech may be appropriate.

Pitch

The pitch of a voice describes how high, like a treble in a choir, or low, like the bass, it sounds. As the hearing deficit associated with age (presbyacusis) tends to affect higher-pitched sound, then a lower pitch may be adopted when speaking to an elderly patient with a hearing problem. This is most effective if combined with a clear enunciation of words, the mouth of the speaker in full view of the listener.
Increasing the volume is rarely appropriate when speaking to patients with hearing difficulties as it tends to distort the sound.

Volume

Altering the volume of the spoken word allows a speaker to give emphasis to particular words or expressions that they might want a patient to remember. It is also a useful technique in maintaining a patient's attention.

Pauses

Analysis of recordings of conversations or of clinical interactions shows that a considerable amount of the time is taken up by silence. Long pauses may be disconcerting and create a distance between the practitioner and patient. If a silence is necessary then a preceding explanation is helpful, for example, "I'm just going to make a few notes now".

Synchrony and pacing

Synchrony is a term to describe the adoption by the practitioner of nonverbal behavior to match or complement that of the patient, so avoiding for example the use of dominant and extrovert body posture when with a particularly timid patient. Pacing describes the movement of the practitioner reflecting that of the patient, for example leaning forward when the patient does. If done carefully then, far from looking like a second-rate mime act, the practitioner may give the impression of understanding and empathy with the patient.

The CLOSER model

A model of good physical attending on the part of a practitioner has been suggested and is summed up by the mnemonic CLOSER (after Ettinger, 1994). This involves the following behaviors:

C Control any distractions and potential interruptions that may interfere with attention.
L Lean forward slightly toward the patient.
O Maintain an open, nondefensive posture and appear relaxed and at ease with the surroundings.
S Face the patient squarely.
E Maintain eye contact as appropriate.
R Respect the patient's personal space and position in the room.

Question strategy: gaining cognitive information

The way a question is asked may significantly affect the response. A question in several parts (compound) may be confusing or daunting for a patient with poor memory or who is inhibited. A leading question, one with an implicit answer, may encourage a less than accurate response. An open question may not allow a very shy patient to give all the facts. For this reason it may be useful to recall the different categories of questions that exist:

- **Open questions** These cannot be answered by a simple "yes" or "no" or a single statement of fact and tend to begin with "what", "when", "where", "why" and "how". These are good scene-setting questions as they allow some freedom of response by the patient. They also allow a good degree of affective assessment of the patient as the way a very open question is answered is often dictated by a patient's emotions, feelings, or prejudices.
- **Closed questions** These tend to follow open questions. They allow only a simple "yes" or "no" or single response and are useful at finding specific information, such as "Is there anyone in your family who has glaucoma?"

Careful use of the above question types aid in controlling a patient's response. A very talkative patient may be curtailed somewhat by closed questioning so that only information of use to the practitioner is given. A very shy or introvert patient may be encouraged to give answers initially to closed questions and, once some confidence has been gained, more open questions may be usefully employed (a so-called "funneling technique").

- **Direct and indirect questions** A direct question may be open or closed and is one where there is very obviously one particular answer. For example, a direct open question might be "Tell me about the types of activity where you use your distance glasses." A direct closed question might be "Do you wear your glasses when driving?" Indirect questions, on the other hand, do not sound like questions at all and often help in the building of trust and rapport between patient and optometrist, for example, "It would appear that you don't really wear your distance glasses. You must have wondered what you were given them for."

- **Compound questions** These are multiple questions, such as "Have you ever been prescribed glasses for driving, or reading, or computer use or for any hobby or occupation?" Such questions are best avoided as not only might they confuse a patient who is unsure as to exactly which of the sequence of questions to answer, but also any response (in this example a simple "yes") may not give a clear idea as to what is being answered.

- **Leading questions** These are questions within which the answer is implicit. An example would be "Your general health is quite good at the moment, isn't it?" It is a technique that may have some use in particularly unresponsive or unforth-coming patients but more often than not tells more about the questioner's viewpoint than the respondent.

- **"Questionnaire" questions** These present the patient with a series of possible responses. An example would be "Does this lens make the letters more clear, less clear or exactly the same as before?" By providing a choice of preset answers, this tech-nique is often useful in the less responsive or introverted patient.

- **Probing questions** This term is often used and tends to describe a sequence of (often closed) questions that gradually give an increasing picture about a particular point.

- **Facilitative questions and statements** These are important encouraging remarks such as "Would you like to continue?" or "Please do go on" which, combined with appropriate nonverbal cues, such as nods and smiles, encourage the patient and instill some confidence in the practitioner's listening ability.

- **Clarifying questions and statements** These are useful in making sure a particular point has been understood correctly. This may be done by the practitioner paraphrasing the points given by the patient and checking that that was what was meant.

A refinement of this is sometimes referred to as the process of reflection whereby a clarifying question may encourage the patient to divulge further information. For example, upon being told that a patient is worried by a symptom, the practitioner might ask "Very worried?" At the end of a sequence of information transfer, whether it be history and symptoms or giving information to the patient, a summary of the information is useful to clarify matters for both the patient and practitioner.

- **Validating questions or statements** These are clarification techniques that go one stage further by implying some inference by the practitioner often gained from nonverbal as well as verbal cues, for example, "Would you like me to explain why it is important to know what medications you use?" This technique is of some use with uncooperative or anxious patients.

- **Confronting questions or statements** These may be the only recourse in a situation where it is necessary to directly confront a situation where further progress may be hindered. An example might be "You seem very angry. Would you tell me why this is so that I can continue the examination?" Obviously such a potentially explosive situation needs careful handling and direct confrontation may not always be appropriate.

It would be foolish to suggest a strict pattern of question type use to be applied to a particular interview ("for a nervous patient use three open then two closed and a questionnaire-type question") and obviously each individual case needs personalised management. Furthermore, the use of speech is difficult to control in such a strict grammatical manner. The point is that, by being aware of the importance of different grammatical constructions, one may, over a period of time, adapt one's interview technique to obtain information more successfully.

The nature of the history and symptoms interview

There are arguments against describing the history and symptoms interview under separate headings relating to the different aspects of a patient, such as their ocular history or their family ocular history and so on. A purely problem-oriented approach would lead the optometrist to ascertain any symptom or reason for attendance and then to ask further questions to shed light on this particular need.

A checklist approach, where one simply asks a set list of questions relating to each of the categories mentioned below, has the advantage of establishing potentially useful baseline data even if some of this is not relevant on the day. For example, to discover a strong family history of glaucoma in the family of a 16-year-old may prove more important later on in the patient's life. A disadvantage, apart from the risk of using time less than efficiently, is the possibility that the optometrist, by dwelling on a fact of no immediate relevance to the matter in hand, such as a patient's medication history, may fail to grasp that the main reason for the patient's attendance is to ask about varifocals. Careful explanation by the optometrist of the need to ask certain facts should prevent this happening.

A sensible approach would appear to be a combination of the two. All relevant baseline information should be established even if not of immediate relevance to the particular problem presenting on the day, but any specific problem needs more probing to elicit its exact nature.

In occasional cases where a patient is apparently reluctant to offer information or questions the relevance of certain questions (typically those about general health issues), it is most useful for the optometrist to explain that, in order to assess the health of the eyes adequately, a bigger picture of the patient's well-being needs to be gained. Eyes are affected by many general health factors.

The questioning is necessarily going to be different for every patient, but a systematic approach helps the optometrist to remember to ask all relevant questions. This should be recorded carefully and clearly, so providing important personal details together with what may be described as a subjective problem list.

One suggested structure for areas to be investigated during the history and symptoms interview now follows.

Reason for attendance

It is generally considered that an appreciation of why the patient has attended for an eye examination should be gained from the outset. Whether it is a routine two-yearly recall or a specific concern regarding a particular problem, all subsequent questions and actions by the practitioner may follow on from this premise. An initial question is usually an open one, that is, one for which there is not a simple yes/no or single statement answer.

"Tell me why you've come to see me today" may elicit more immediate information from the patient than "Do you have a particular problem with your eyes?", though the latter may be appropriate as a follow-up question in some circumstances or in cases of poor response from the patient.

Current ocular and optical status

Details about the patient's current vision, correction, any symptoms are elicited. As this is a more specific line of questioning where some essential facts need to be established, closed questions with one specific answer may be appropriate. Furthermore, while the practitioner should be aware of the pitfall of sounding as though they are reading a list of pre-written questions, it is often important to ask questions of a patient to rule out certain possibilities. For example it is common practice to establish that the patient has not experienced photopsia, but unless this is asked the patient who has reported no particular symptom cannot be assumed to have not experienced photopsia.

A typical list of initial questions might include the following, most of which may then lead on to more specific questions:

- **Do you see well in the distance?** (examples may be given, such as driving, television and so on)
- **Do you see near objects well?** (usually reference to reading ability is made)

Any blur should be qualified further in terms of distance, near or both, which eye (or both), onset and duration, and so on.

- **Do you currently wear any vision correction?** (what type, standard of vision with correction, condition of correction, and so on)
- **Do you experience any…?**

This last question may allow one to find out whether a patient has experience of a whole range of symptoms. To reproduce a list invites the criticism that it is encouraging a practitioner to read out automaton-like a list of potential symptoms and that a better approach would be to adapt one's individual questioning to the specific needs of the patient. However, relevant symptoms might include:

Headaches
Further questioning here might ascertain:

- Which part of the head?
- Both sides or one?
- Nature of the pain (sharp, throbbing, dull, cluster and so on)
- Associated nausea and vomiting
- Associated visual disturbance (migraine as opposed to possible ischemic incident)
- Medication being taken for headache
- Association with any task, visual or possibly other activity

Eye pain
- Constant or intermittent
- Nature of the pain (severe or otherwise)
- Associated with eye movement

Floaters
- Location in view
- Size
- Moves with the eye
- Solid or web-like
- Associations, such as trauma

Flashes of light
- Persistent or transient
- Associated with onset of floaters (see previous list)
- One or both eyes

Itching, redness, soreness, tearing, burning, etc.
- One or both eyes
- Any associations (outdoors, light, season and so on)
- Nature of any discharge

Double vision
- Double as opposed to blurred (many patients may be confused by the difference so the practitioner must be careful to help in the distinction)
- Monocular or binocular
- Vertical or horizontal

This list, for the reasons already outlined, is not exhaustive and each patient should be taken individually. The follow-up questions usefully allow the practitioner to qualify individual symptoms.

So the general pattern so far has been of an initial open questioning followed by more specific, possibly closed questions about presenting symptoms, affirmative responses being further probed to gain more specific detail. The overall pattern of initial open questioning followed by successive increasingly closed questions is sometimes called a funnel approach. A list of questions of similar form or depth is sometimes called a tunnel approach or technique. The probing questions appropriate for symptoms are summarized in Table 2.1.

Patient ocular history

Details regarding any history of:
- Last eye examination
- Optical correction (type, when and how long worn, condition)
- Injury or trauma

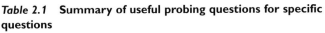

Table 2.1 Summary of useful probing questions for specific questions

History	When was it first noticed, had it before?
Onset	Sudden or gradual?
Timing	Specifically when does it happen?
Causative factors	Does anything start or stop it?
Duration	How long does it last?
Frequency	Constant or intermittent?
Associations	Other symptoms with it?
Change	Getting better or worse?
Other	Does your GP know? Family history?

- Surgery, orthoptic or refractive treatment
- Known eye disease or "squint"

The term "squint" should always be qualified as, together with astigmatism and "lazy eye", it is open to misinterpretation. It will, however, be used instead of "strabismus" throughout the remainder of this book as it is the term most likely to be understood by the patient.

Family ocular history

Details regarding any family members with:
- Visual problems (high myopia, amblyopia and so on)
- "Squints"
- Eye diseases (glaucoma, nystagmus and many others)

Patient general medical history

This is one particular area where the use of a leading question may confuse the issue. To ask of a patient "Is your health good at the moment?" may elicit a definite "Yes, thank you" from a patient who has just been through a period of poor health which has recently stabilized. An insulin-dependent diabetic may feel in the best of health. More useful approaches might include:

- How is your health at the moment?
- Do you have to visit your doctor for any reason?
- Are you taking any medication at present (or have been recently)?
- Are you being treated for diabetes or hypertension?
- Are you being treated or investigated for any general health problems?

With regard to medication, the more detail the better and it is often considered good practice to look at drug bottles, prescriptions or any literature the patient may possess. Some indication as to patient compliance, for example use of glaucoma drops or control of sugar levels in diabetes, may be obtained through careful questioning here.

With some conditions, such as hypertension, further questioning may be appropriate to ensure that the patient is being monitored regularly and that they are aware of the importance of adequate control of their condition.

With diabetes in particular, some more detail may be of direct relevance to the optometrist and may influence the nature of the subsequent correspondence with the general practitioner. Follow-up questions might include:

- Duration of the disease.
- Nature of the disease (Type 1 or 2).
- Nature of the control and whether this has changed, and whether it is stable.
- Who monitors the condition and if other eye examinations are included.
- When was the last medical check and when will the next one be?

Family medical history

Any family history of hypertension, stroke or diabetes (and type) may be of importance.

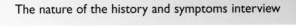
Lifestyle and occupation details

This information may arise during the above questioning. Indeed the presenting problem in many eye examinations may be directly related to problems in the workplace or driving or carrying out a hobby. Asking about the nature of a patient's work is more useful than just knowing a job title, which may be misleading. Use of a computer may lead onto a whole host of further questions. The need to drive may influence one's final consideration of results as there are obvious legal implications here. The practitioner may be able to infer the possible requirement for safety spectacles or advice relating to eye health and safety.

A good concluding question might be "Is there anything else about your eyes or vision which concerns you?" or "Is there anything else about your eyes or health that I should know?" This should fill in any missing detail so that the practical examination may begin with a detailed knowledge of the patient's ocular state.

The problem with drafting a list such as this, on top of tempting a wholesale reading out of a checklist to a patient, is that any comprehensive list seems to be quite daunting. The fact that a skilled practitioner may be able to elicit all the relevant information mentioned above in a perfectly acceptable time is partly due to correct sequencing of questions and the appropriate combination of open and closed and other types of questioning. This is generally done without conscious thought and is certainly a skill that improves with practice.

3
Vision and acuity

Visual acuity and vision

Visual acuity is a measurement of a patient's ability to resolve detail and usually involves directing a patient to identify targets at a set distance which are of ever decreasing size and typically of high contrast until they can no longer be identified. The recognition of high-contrast targets at the highest spatial frequency as described is useful for standardized assessment but is not representative of the visual environment within which the patient lives and hence will not truly represent the patient's visual ability. The unaided visual acuity (usually called the vision) is useful in estimating refractive error before assessment and represents important baseline data where a patient does not use, or perhaps does not need to use, their correction all the time.

The acuity with their current correction is known as the habitual visual acuity and the resultant visual acuity after refraction and full correction of the current refractive error is known as the optimal visual acuity. It is essential for an optometrist to note both the vision and habitual visual acuity prior to any clinical assessment in case of any legal action taken as a result of the examination. Both monocular and binocular acuity should be noted as there may be a discrepancy, such as when a nystagmus patient shows significant acuity improvement when in the binocular state.

Although there are several ways to specify target size on test charts, the most widely used system was introduced by Snellen in 1862. He assumed that the "average" eye could just read a letter if the thickness of the limbs and the spaces between them subtended 1 minute of arc at the eye. Thus the letter E would subtend 5 minutes of arc vertically. Snellen notation requires the acuity allowing the eye to resolve such a letter to be noted down as a fraction with the viewing distance (usually in meters and commonly 6 m) over the distance at which such a target would subtend 5 minutes of arc vertically. Thus at 6 m a 6/6 letter subtends 5 minutes of arc vertically, a 6/12 letter 10 minutes and a 6/60 letter 50 minutes. The Snellen fraction may also be written as a decimal, for example 6/6 = 1, 6/12 = 0.5 and 6/60 = 0.1.

Table 3.1 **The relationship between different acuity scales**

Snellen	Decimal	MAR	LogMAR
6/60	0.10	10	1.000
6/24	0.25	4	0.602
6/12	0.50	2	0.301
6/6	1.00	1	0.000
6/4	1.50	0.667	−0.176

An alternative is to record the minimum angle of resolution (MAR). The MAR relates to the resolution required to resolve the elements of a letter. Thus 6/6 equates to an MAR of 1 minute of arc, 6/12 to an MAR of 2 and 6/60 to 10. The logMAR score is the $\log_{10}$ of the MAR so is 0 for 6/6 and 1 for 6/60. This means that targets smaller than the 6/6 letters, which would be expected to be resolved by a young healthy adult, would carry a negative score value. Some acuity values are shown in different notation in Table 3.1.

LogMAR notation

Though Snellen notation is still in widespread use, there are criticisms of the standard Snellen chart as shown in Figure 3.1. There are fewer large letters so providing an unequal challenge to those with reduced vision, the letter spacing reduces leading to crowding on lower lines, the line separation is not regular so the challenge changes on reading down the chart, which means that moving charts to different working distances alters the demand on acuity. LogMAR charts, such as the Bailey–Lovie chart shown in Figure 3.2, address some of these shortcomings by having spacing between letters on each line related to the width of the letters and between rows relating to the height of the letters, and an equal number of letters on each line. This provides a constant task as the patient reads down the chart, allowing it to be viewed at different working distances and the acuity to be more easily correlated. Such charts have been found to give greater repeatability of

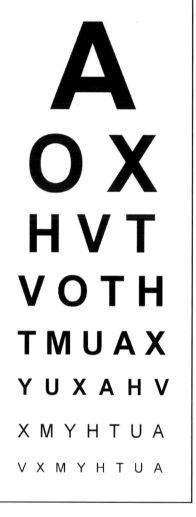

Figure 3.1 The standard Snellen chart

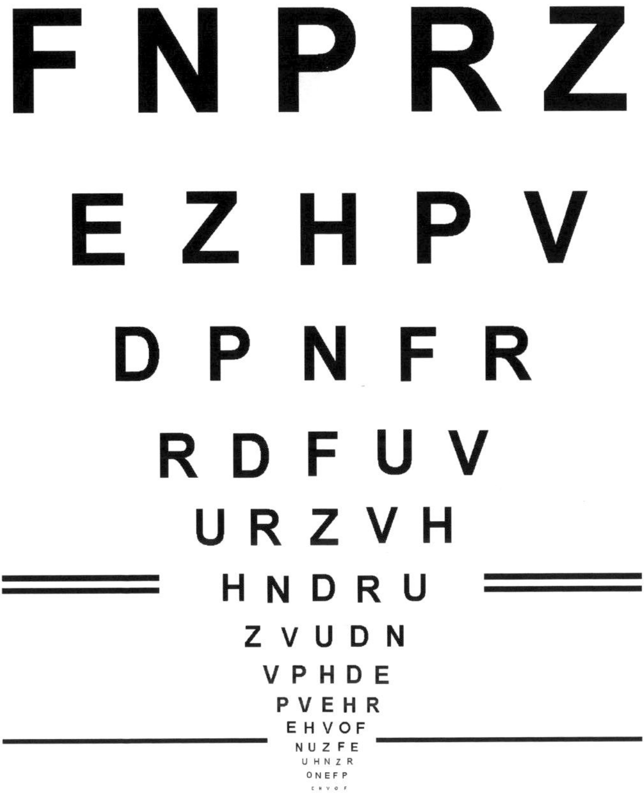

F N P R Z

E Z H P V

D P N F R

R D F U V

U R Z V H

═══ H N D R U ═══

Z V U D N

V P H D E

P V E H R

E H V O F

N U Z F E

U H N Z R

O N E F P

Figure 3.2 The Bailey–Lovie LogMAR chart

measurement and be more sensitive to detect interocular acuity differences.

LogMAR scores may be noted on record cards either relating to the smallest target line size seen or using the Visual Acuity Rating where 0.02 is added for every letter missed on the line. So where a patient just manages the 6/6 line and no more, they are scored as 0. If they miss two letters on this line they are scored as 0.04. Until this notation becomes universally accepted, Snellen notation is still appropriate for referrals and inter-professional communication. Most logMAR charts in use are calibrated for a working distance of 4 m.

When one has to reduce the distance, for example for a low-vision patient, it is useful to remember to add 0.3 to the score for every time the distance is halved. For example the ability to read the top line at 4 m would be scored as acuity of 1.0. At 2 m, this would be scored as 1.3.

Where letter recognition is not possible, for example with small children or patients of different literacy, a whole range of picture and line targets are available. Some require identification, others matching of targets with a separate key card. For the very young, the use of gratings of different spatial frequency next to blank targets may be presented to see if the infant's attention is directed to the grating. Such preferential-looking tests have been found to show good repeatability in pediatric assessment.

Contrast sensitivity testing

There is a strong argument for assessing the contrast sensitivity of patients during a routine eye examination. However, because of the relative difficulty in assessing changes in quality of vision during the refraction and correction process, together with variations in recording of results, the assessment is rarely included in all but specialized routines (such as the assessment of the visually impaired).

The ability to resolve targets varies significantly with the contrast of the target. The visual world a patient inhabits is one of varying target size and contrast and, furthermore, diseases affecting vision may affect the ability to resolve these targets in a selective manner. Therefore the use of high-contrast targets for acuity testing has been criticized as non-representative of the visual world and less than sensitive at reflecting visual reduction due to disease. If a patient is shown a sine-wave grating of a constant spatial frequency, as shown in Figure 3.3, their ability to resolve the grating reduces as the contrast is reduced until a point is reached when it can no longer be resolved. This point, the contrast threshold (the reciprocal of which is called the contrast sensitivity), is different for different spatial frequencies and the plot of the threshold values against spatial frequency is described as the contrast sensitivity function (CSF), as shown in Figure 3.4.

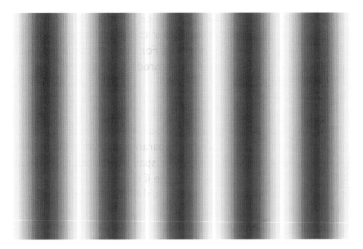

Figure 3.3   A sine-wave grating

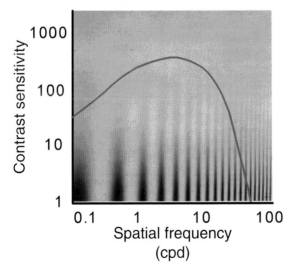

Figure 3.4   Contrast sensitivity function

Snellen acuity relates to the resolution of a high-contrast target of maximum spatial frequency and is therefore represented as the cut-off point on the horizontal axis on this curve. This is sensitive to conditions affecting mainly high spatial frequencies, such as refractive error, but less sensitive if lower spatial frequencies are affected, as with cataract, corneal disturbance and contact lens wear.

Increasingly clinicians are using targets of different contrast to assess the influence upon acuity. LogMAR charts are available in different contrasts, so assessing the patient's ability to resolve increasing spatial frequencies at a given contrast value. Computerized acuity charts, such as the City2000 shown in Figure 3.5, allow any contrast value to be preset.

Other charts, such as the Pelli–Robson, use a constant letter size (approximating to one cycle per degree if viewed at 1 m) and gradually reducing contrast as the chart is read by the patient. In theory, varying the working distance would allow the whole

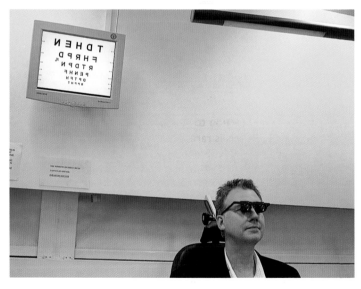

Figure 3.5 Computerized acuity chart (e.g. the City2000)

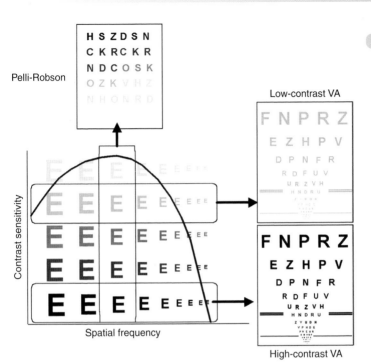

Figure 3.6 Relating high- and low-contrast visual acuity and Pelli–Robson contrast sensitivity to the contrast sensitivity function

contrast sensitivity function to be assessed with a Pelli–Robson chart, but in practice this is rarely needed as high- and low-contrast acuity scores combined with contrast sensitivity at 1 m with a Pelli–Robson is usually sufficient to suggest any visual compromise. The relationship between the charts and the CSF is shown in Figure 3.6.

Routine

At the outset of the assessment the optometrist should establish acuity and vision, and the following list represents a few important points to bear in mind when doing so:

- Binocular followed by monocular acuity is useful. The binocular acuity is occasionally different to the monocular (for example much better in many nystagmus patients). Also this order allows an assessment of acuity prior to the breakdown of a less stable binocular state once an occluder is introduced.
- The acuity with current spectacles is useful as it represents the patient's actual experience. It is important therefore to simulate as closely as possible the typical viewing conditions for the patient (usually with the room lights on).
- If one eye is known to have poorer vision, this should be assessed first to minimize any learning of targets.
- An occluder should be used and checked for correct placement. Use of hands should be avoided as often the patient may see through a gap between fingers not apparent to anyone else.
- Any indication of the quality of the acuity should be noted together with the notation for the minimum target size seen (for example "blurred 6/12-1", or "6/48 viewed eccentrically")
- For distance acuity, note should be made of the correction being worn and its condition.
- For near acuity, a target distance relating to the patient's everyday experience (computer or reading distance) should be adopted. For near visions, the distance at which the best vision is achieved gives some clues about the uncorrected refractive error and this should be noted.
- When uncorrected vision is poor, it is better to attempt some sort of quantification than to rely upon imprecise statements such as "count fingers". If the patient is mobile they may be moved closer to the chart, though a movable chart is preferable (as long as the appropriate adjustment is made to the acuity measurement).

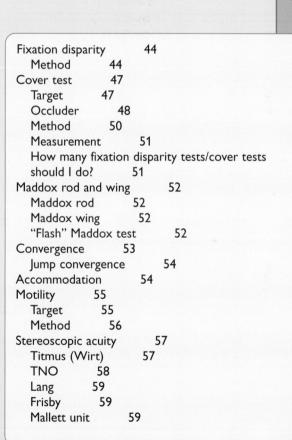

4
Binocular assessment

The assessment of binocular function is often one of the weaker areas of a routine, if observation of candidates in the PQE is any guide. Tests are done for no clearly logical reason, often because they always have been, and in an order that defeats the object of the testing. Binocular vision seems to be one of those areas that practitioners shy away from, and students often take an instant dislike to. Many retests and subsequent remakes of spectacles are the result of a practitioner overlooking the effects of a change of prescription on the binocular status of the patient.

It would be useful to define what it is we are trying to find out:

- Does the patient have a squint or a phoria?
- If they have a phoria, is it compensated?
- If they have a binocular problem, is it going to need referral or management?

Tests of motor function can be divided into those "binocular" tests that maintain fusion (e.g. fixation disparity) and those that dissociate the eyes (e.g. cover test, Maddox rod). As a general principle, binocular tests should always precede dissociation tests. In practice, this is often reversed and frequently patients are tested for fixation disparity having been thoroughly dissociated before, and in some cases during, the test. The odd false-positive might be expected in these cases.

Fixation disparity

Method

The fixation disparity test is often performed in such a way as to render it worthless. Even the wording of the instructions and questions given to the patient can affect the chances of finding a fixation disparity, particularly in children and the more literal-minded adult.

- This test should ideally precede any dissociation test.
- Binocular vision should be stabilized, by reading a line of letters or words before the assessment of fixation disparity.

This is particularly important if the patient has been
dissociated recently, and they always will have. Taking
monocular acuities, retinoscopy, ophthalmoscopy and so
on will all disrupt the binocular status.
- It should be remembered that the polarized visor used
significantly reduces light levels and illumination should be
adjusted accordingly.
- Before applying the visor, the patient should be asked "Are the
two red (or green) lines exactly in line with each other or are
they out of line?" It is surprising how often a patient will
report displacement of the lines even without the visor.
Are they trustworthy observers? Do you want to prescribe
on their subjective response?
- Having established that the patient isn't likely to lead you
astray, repeat the previous question. Leading questions should
be avoided, especially when dealing with children.
- If they are out of line, ask the patient "Which one is out of line
with the X?" You should know before you start the test which
line is seen by which eye. If you can't remember it from last
time, it's simply a matter of looking at the target through the
visor yourself. Even if you think you can remember, have a
look anyway, because it is not unknown for the polarization
of the visor not to match that of the Mallett unit at distance
or near or both, especially if the visor is a replacement. If
both eyes can see both bars, nobody will have a fixation
disparity. Under no circumstances cover up one of the patient's
eyes and say "Which line can you see now?" This will result in
an unwanted dissociation (Figure 4.1).
- Then ask "Is it to the left or to the right?" OR "Is it toward
me or away from me?" With children, the latter question may
be more sensible, as they do tend to mix up their lefts and
rights on occasion.
- The minimum prism (to the nearest 1/2Δ) or alteration in the
spherical element of the Rx which aligns the polarized lines
should be noted.

When assessing fixation disparity for near, don't be restricted
to one target position. Many patients read or look at computer

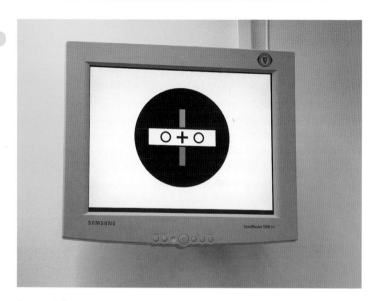

Figure 4.1 A distance fixation disparity target

screens in a variety of positions. Many patients have "A" and "V" patterns and it doesn't take long to check if the patient is still compensated when the eyes are elevated or depressed.

Until you have done a cover test, you won't necessarily know what the fixation disparity findings mean. No slip found on a patient with a phoria would indicate that the phoria is compensated, at least for the moment, but the same finding on a strabismic subject would indicate harmonious anomalous retinal correspondence. Small degrees of slip usually point toward an uncompensated phoria, especially if there are symptoms, but a larger slip may be associated with microtropia.

Sometimes the slip seems to vary at random, and the markers may oscillate across the neutral point. This is indicative of binocular instability. The condition is associated with uncompensated heterophoria and the fusional reserves tend to be low. In general, if you keep adding small amounts of prism or sphere, the slip will stabilize.

The cover test is essential, being the only way to tell squints and
phorias apart. It can also be used to estimate or measure the
direction and size of the deviation and to indicate whether a phoria
is compensated or not. There is a certain amount of confusion
about the cover test, partly arising because it tends to be taught in
a module labeled "binocular vision" and often based on orthoptic
practice rather than the needs of a routine eye examination. While
there is considerable overlap, the two have different goals and
requirements (also refer to Binocular Vision by Bruce Evans). In a
routine eye examination we are screening a normal population
for those individuals whose motor or sensory status requires
intervention. In the hospital eye service, there is a greater need
to classify and quantify so that the effects of treatment may be
recorded. As this is a book about routine eye examination, the
approach will be biased toward that.

Target

- The target should be accommodative (that is, one small enough
  for the hypermetrope to employ enough accommodation to
  overcome their ametropia and hence reveal any eso-movement),
  so use a letter slightly larger than the acuity of the worst eye.
  If the target is too small, the maintenance of accurate fixation
  is difficult. The patient may narrow the palpebral fissure to see
  better, making observation of the eyes difficult. Occasionally
  ciliary spasm might be triggered.
- If the acuity of the worst eye is below 6/18 a spotlight may be
  used. Note that this is a non-accommodative target. The reason
  for using it is that the angular subtense of letters larger than
  6/18 is large enough to significantly distort the results, particularly when looking at small vertical elements. However, many
  practitioners find that there is still more eso-deviation when a
  letter target is used. If in doubt, use both.
- The position of the target is important, particularly at near.
  The cover test should be performed with fixation at a distance

and position that is relevant to the current patient and their habitual visual environment. There is occasionally a tendency to perform the near cover test with the eyes level, in the same position that they were in when fixating a distant target. This is fine if you want to compare distance and near deviations while removing any variability that an A or V pattern would induce, in other words, if you are trying to classify the deviation accurately. However, we are generally trying to find out what is happening while the patient goes about their daily business.

- When performing the near cover test, it is a good idea to quickly check if there are any significant variations with elevation and depression of gaze. Multiple positions of fixation may be useful to investigate incomitancy.

- When examining myopic patients without their spectacles it should be remembered that unaided distance vision below 6/60 does not mean that a non-accommodative target should be used at near. Many myopes habitually read without spectacles at a non-standard distance, and most will be able to fixate an accommodative target for the near cover test. This applies to myopic presbyopes too.

Occluder

- The occluder may be opaque or translucent. The latter allows us to observe eye movements behind the cover (Figure 4.2b) and is particularly helpful when trying to see dissociated vertical deviations. The use of fingers, thumbs, hands, etc., should be avoided as adequate dissociation may not be achieved.

- Translucency or a white back is an asset, causing fewer pupil reactions which can be distracting when looking at small deviations (Figure 4.2b).

- Opaque occluders should be wide enough to allow them to be angled so as to allow observation of the eye under the cover (Figure 4.2a), while maintaining proper dissociation.

- Occluders should ideally have no sharp corners. In most respects other than this a frame rule makes a good occluder, but there is an outside chance of catching a lively patient in the eye with it.

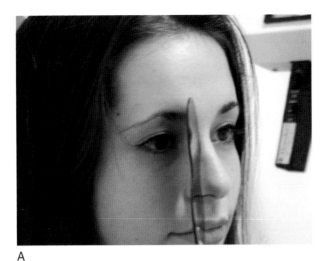

A

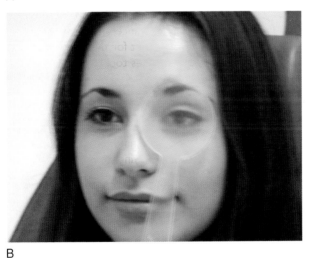

B

Figure 4.2 **(A)** An opaque occluder needs to be angled to allow viewing of the eye behind. **(B)** A translucent cover allowing the eye movement to be seen while still maintaining dissociation

Method

- The cover should be held over the eye for 5 seconds, which is rather longer than initially feels right. Less may result in incomplete dissociation and an underestimation of the deviation. It should be remembered that repeated testing may increase the deviation through fatigue.
- The cover should be held close to the eye or dissociation may be incomplete.
- Cover the right eye and observe the left. If it moves to take up fixation there is a squint. If it doesn't move there is either no squint or a microtropia with identity.
- Uncover the right eye, still watching the left. If it moves now, two things are possible. If it moved to take up fixation when you covered the right eye, it's a squint and it's now moving back into its customary position. If there was no movement of the left eye when you covered the right, you are seeing a "Hering movement" and the patient has central suppression in the left eye.
- If no movement is seen in the left eye, cover the right eye again but watch the right eye under the cover this time. If it moves out, the patient has an exophoria. If it moves in, they have an esophoria. If it goes down, they have a hypophoria. Should it go up, they may have a hyperphoria or a dissociated vertical deviation, or both. If it's a right hyperphoria the left eye will move down when it is covered, and back up again when it is uncovered.
- Uncover the right eye, watch the right eye. It should be seen to move back to fixation. If it doesn't, the patient may have dissociated and broken down to a squint.
- Repeat the above, covering the left eye.

The **objective alternate cover test** is often employed to investigate phorias. If you are dissociating the patient properly during the cover/uncover test, it will add nothing that you don't already know. If you are finding a different deviation with the alternate cover test, you aren't dissociating for long enough on the cover/uncover test.

The **subjective alternate cover ("phi") test** is a different matter. This can detect deviations that are too small to be seen by the practitioner (typically less than 1Δ). One of the recurrent myths in optometry is the one that says that deviations below 4Δ cannot be detected by the human eye. This is nonsense, and the easiest way to prove this is to observe a subject successively fixating test chart letters of known separation. These are rarely of much significance if horizontal, but small vertical deviations are surprisingly common and may be a pointer toward incomitancy. To do this, alternate the cover between the two eyes, and ask the patient if the target is moving at all. If it is, determine whether it moves in the same direction as the cover, which indicates exophoria, or in the opposite direction, as it would with an esophoric patient. If there is a vertical movement, the Maddox rod is indicated.

Measurement

This may be achieved with loose prisms or a prism bar, but is rarely necessary in routine examination. Estimation is accurate enough with practice unless surgery is contemplated (unlikely in routine practice). To practice, a tangent screen is useful, but not essential if you are able to observe a subject fixating successively two targets of known angular separation. At 6 m, separation of 12 cm corresponds to 2Δ (this is about the width of the 6/9 line on a standard Snellen chart), 24 cm corresponds to 4Δ and so on.

How many fixation disparity tests/cover tests should I do?

It depends what you need to know. In general, you want to know if any correction that the patient is currently wearing is allowing the patient comfortable vision, so checking both fixation disparity and cover test at any fixation distance relevant to the patient (including VDU distance in many cases) would seem a good idea. You may also need to know what happens without the correction. It is usually worth checking for A and V patterns when you have the patient fixating a near target. If you change the prescription significantly during the routine, you should check if the change has affected the binocular status. Remember that even small changes in refraction can affect ocular motor balance significantly, so even increasing a reading addition by half a diopter can induce an uncompensated exophoria if care is not taken.

Maddox rod and wing

Maddox rod

This may be used to measure the deviation using either prisms or a tangent scale. Correlation with cover test results is poor, probably due to the abnormal visual environment generated by the Maddox rod. It should also be remembered that the test uses a non accommodative target. It is said to measure the "total phoria", though as long is the patient is alive this is not so. It also generates numbers without requiring any observation skills. It is useful to identify and measure small deviations (particularly vertical ones) and to investigate incomitancies. In routine refraction its use is rarely justified since it adds no new information to that found with the cover test and it usually seems to constitute a box-filling exercise.

Maddox wing

This is a convenient test for measurement of the deviation, but correlation with cover test results is poor and correlation of either with symptoms is bad. Is the cover test is always done, it is questionable whether this test yields any essential information most of the time. The target is set at 30 cm, which is too short for anyone over 5 ft, and the scale is a poor accommodative target.

"Flash" Maddox test

This is basically a cover test which uses the tangent scales of the Maddox rod or wing to measure the deviation, as an alternative to prism measurement. The eye fixating the streak, or the arrow of the wing test, is covered. The patient is instructed to tell you which number the streak or arrow is pointing to immediately after you remove the cover. This is probably the most useful way to use Maddox tests and it has been used in research (e.g. by North and Henson, 1981, to investigate prism adaptation).

Convergence

- The RAF rule is the usual tool but any thin vertical line will do, as will a single letter on a budgie stick. The end of the instrument nearest to the eyes should be supported by the patient to ensure that it cannot slip and catch the eye. Care should be taken that the rule is angled slightly downward rather than perpendicular to the face or higher as the eyes usually look slightly down when converging, and most patients find convergence easier with some depression of the eyes (Figure 4.3). However, there

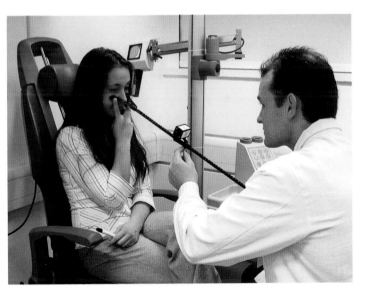

Figure 4.3 The RAF rule should be used in a downward position to maximize convergence

are exceptions to both of these statements. VDU operators may need to converge with their eyes level or elevated, and those with A patterns may be happier in this position.

- The target is moved slowly toward the patient and the patient is asked to report when the target goes double (normally 8–10 cm). The target is then withdrawn until recovery occurs (normally 10–15 cm). The near point is often more remote in tall patients or those with long working distances. This test activates both voluntary and reflex convergence.

- The practitioner should watch the eyes, rather than relying on the patient to report diplopia. Sometimes convergence breaks but the patient does not report diplopia. This may simply be down to wandering attention, but it could also indicate suppression. The eye doesn't necessarily always deviate outward. Patients with esophoria and a high AC/A ration will over-converge.

- The near point of convergence should be recorded in centimeters, along with which eye deviated and in which direction. If the patient does not report diplopia when dissociated, this should also be noted.

Jump convergence

Jump convergence is useful, especially in those who need to change fixation frequently. The patient is asked to fixate in turn on distant and near targets and to report any diplopia. Voluntary convergence is almost exclusively activated by this test.

Accommodation

This will be discussed in Chapter 9 which examines near corrections, though it is frequently investigated along with near point of convergence.

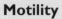

Motility

Target

The ideal target is a pen-torch, used unfocused, and preferably not too bright, held in the way shown in Figure 4.4. Too bright a torch may cause spontaneous dissociation, especially in exophores, and avoidable discomfort. Paradoxically, cheap and nasty pen-torches obtainable from market traders are often the best, and they are cheap enough to be lost without pain. The pen-torch allows us to see a reflex on the cornea which may help to decide if both eyes are fixating the target. This is particularly useful when the visual axis of one of the eyes is intercepted by the patient's nose. Under such circumstances we are effectively performing a cover test and the patient's phoria will be

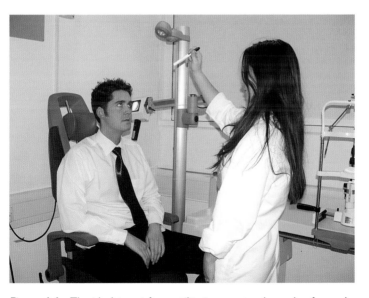

Figure 4.4 The ideal target for motility is a pen-torch, used unfocused, and preferably not too bright

expressed. Unless we know that one of the eyes cannot see the target it is possible that we might misinterpret the deviation as being due to an incomitancy, rather than the relationship between accommodation and convergence. However, some practitioners do seem to carry this to extremes, turning off the main room lights in order to see the reflex better. It's true you can see the reflex very well, but little else is discernible. Keep the lights on, you are less likely to miss something important.

Method

- Instruct the patient to follow the target and report any diplopia or pain.
- The practitioner should rely on observation of the patient's eyes rather than patient reports as the patient might be suppressing.
- The pattern used is of little consequence provided that it is methodical. A "star" pattern is typically used (Figure 4.5) but the "H" pattern or its variants are equally effective.

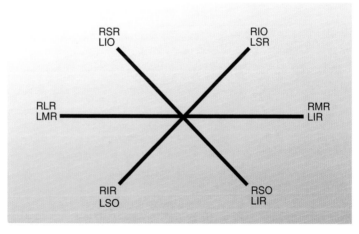

Figure 4.5 Diagnostic positions of gaze

- Move the target slowly or you will not be able to interpret the movement of the eyes.
- If you think there might be an incomitancy present but it isn't an obvious one, base your diagnosis on the cover test in different positions of gaze rather than simple observation of the moving eyes. It is far too easy to see what you want to see, especially when under stress (exams, for instance).
- All eight diagnostic positions of gaze should be investigated, the straight up and down positions being used to look for A- and V-syndromes rather than any specific muscle anomaly.
- The eyelids should also be observed as a narrowing of the palpebral fissure may indicate the presence of Duane's syndrome.
- Voluntary movements (as opposed to the pursuit movements used in motility) may be checked during ophthalmoscopy. It is possible for one to be normal and the other not.

You should always write something down in the records.

- If there is no anomaly write FULL AND NORMAL.
- If an anomaly is present, record which eye is affected, and in which position(s) of gaze.
- If you can, work out which muscle is palsied, and write it down.

Stereoscopic acuity

This is an indication of binocularity. Where visual acuities are good and equal, stereoscopic acuity should be good, even in pre-school children (though with these patients it may be more difficult to demonstrate). Poor stereoscopic acuity in patients with good visual acuity is indicative of poorly compensated ocular motor balance. Useful tests include:

Titmus (Wirt)

This is supposed to be performed at 40 cm but the actual testing distance depends on the length of the patient's arms (Figure 4.6).

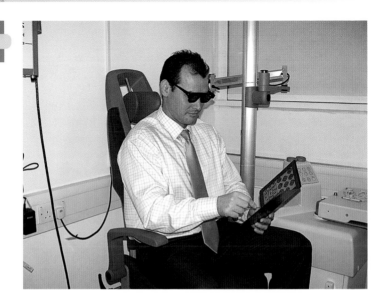

Figure 4.6 Titmus (Wirt) test

The patient wears polarizing spectacles. It can measure stereoscopic acuity up to 40 seconds of arc. It also features more gross tests for children (the "animals" go down to 100 seconds) but many quite young children can be tested with the main "rings". Those new to the test seem to work their way through the fly and animals just because they have a child sitting in their chair. The gross tests are not compulsory if the patient can do the rings. It is important not to let the patient see the targets without the polarizing visor as monocular cues are rather obvious on the first two rings and the animals.

TNO

This is used at approximately 40 cm with the patient wearing red and green goggles. It can measure stereoscopic acuity up to 15 seconds (but more usually 30 seconds) of arc. There are also some gross tests for children.

Lang

This is a more gross test, designed to be a screening device for young children. The pictures go from 1200 seconds to 550 seconds of arc on the Lang I card, and from 600 seconds to 200 seconds on the Lang II. Failure indicates the presence of a clinically significant anomaly which should be followed up.

Frisby

This consists of random-dot patterns on plastic slabs of varying thicknesses, which should be viewed against (and not too close to) a blank surface. Parallax clues are a problem unless the patient's head is stationary and the test is difficult to explain to under-fives.

Mallett unit

This should be used in near darkness and relies on a degree of patient understanding and compliance often not possible. For this reason, it is probably only worth using if no other stereotest is available, as patients tend to dissociate while using it.

5
Pupil assessment

Pupil reflex assessment

The response of the iris to light levels and with accommodation is a result of a neural reflex pathway that involves the iris, retina, visual pathway, midbrain, and parasympathetic and sympathetic innervation of the eye. As such, clinical assessment of the pupil response to light elicits important information about the health of all these structures.

The pupillary reflex pathway is shown in Figure 5.1. If a pen-torch is presented to one eye, the pupil will constrict (the direct reflex) as will that of the other eye (the consensual reflex). Both will constrict when a patient changes gaze from a distant target to a near one (the near reflex). Ambient lighting should

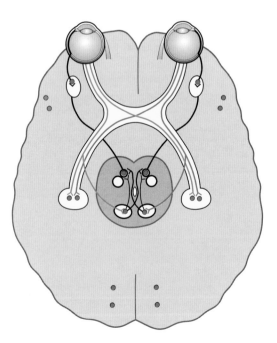

Figure 5.1 The pupillary reflex pathway

be reduced to exaggerate the resting pupil diameter but be of sufficient levels to allow easy viewing of the pupil, particularly in patients with very dark irises. Disruption of the afferent pathway, which may be caused by damage to the retina, optic nerve, chiasma, tract or superior brachium, will result in the loss or reduction of the direct and consensual reflexes. As the damage is often to only some of the pupillary fibers, there may well be a reduction in the pupil response that is only detectable when compared with the normal response; this is described as a relative afferent papillary defect (RAPD) and needs to be detected by the optometrist. This may also be found in patients with a very dense unilateral cataract as light scatter from the opacity may give an enhanced pupil response which appears as an RAPD in the contralateral eye. Some practitioners grade the RAPD by holding varying density filters before the normal eye until the contralateral direct reflex overrides the normal consensual reflex. With conditions where vision loss cannot obviously be traced to ocular signs, for example retrobulbar neuritis, it is essential to investigate anomalous pupil responses.

Damage to the efferent pathway will result in unequal pupil size (anisocoria) and needs to be distinguished from physiological anisocoria, the presence of different pupil sizes not related to any underlying disease process.

Physiological anisocoria

Around one-fifth of people have different pupil sizes, usually less than 0.5 mm difference in diameter. This physiological variation is confirmed by the equal response of the uneven pupils to light stimuli. An easy way to check whether anisocoria is physiological is to measure the two pupils in light and then dark conditions. It is also worth confirming that the difference, if large enough to be noticed, has been known about for a length of time rather than only recently. Generally, physiological anisocoria tends to be small (less than 1 mm), but long-standing larger differences may also be physiological.

Method

- A typical sequence would be to assess the direct and consensual light reflexes for each eye, then to look for an RAPD and finally to assess the near reflex. The latter need not be included in every case as there is no single disease process where the near reflex alone is lost. However, where the direct reflex has been disrupted, the presence of a near reflex is important as part of the diagnosis of Argyll–Robertson pupil. This condition is due to midbrain damage such as occurs in congenital syphilis, and the pupil reflexes resulting were memorably compared by the novelist John Irving to those of a prostitute: accommodating but not able to react directly.
- It is important to establish the best background lighting to best assess pupils and this will vary from patient to patient. A dimmer switch for the consulting room main lights is useful here. The lights should be dim enough to enhance pupil dilation prior to introducing the pen-torch light while bright enough to still allow the consensual reflex to be seen without the pen-torch. So darker irises tend to need more background lighting than paler irises.
- After directing the patient to fixate upon a distance letter target, a bright pen-torch or direct ophthalmoscope light (without too much spread of beam) should be moved in front of one eye from the temporal side of the patient's head (Figure 5.2). A cheap pen-torch is usually all the special equipment required here, though keeping it to within a few centimeters from the target eye will help prevent light spread to the opposite eye. Once in front of one eye, a smooth and obvious constriction should be noted matched by one in the opposite eye. This should be repeated at least three times to look for any gradual reduction in reflex which may indicate an abnormality. Each time the light is removed, a direct and a consensual dilation should also be noticed. The same should be repeated for the opposite eye. As mentioned above, the absence of a direct reflex necessitates the investigation of a near reflex.

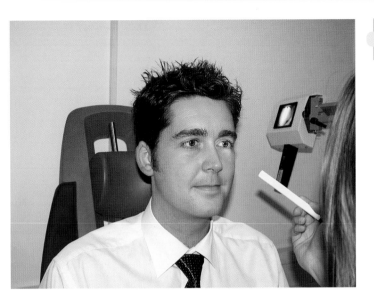

Figure 5.2 A bright pen-torch or direct ophthalmoscope should be moved in front of one eye from the temporal side of the patient's head

- When the light is held in front of one eye for 3 seconds and then moved across to the opposite eye for a further 3 seconds, then back to the first and so on, a sequence of bilateral equal constrictions should be observed. In the case of damage to the afferent pathway (as with, for example, retrobulbar neuritis), the affected eye will show a dilation when the light is moved in front of it from the opposite healthy eye. This is because the consensual reflex from the opposite eye is stronger than the direct response in the affected eye (that is, the afferent signal is present, but defective relative to the other side).
- Most practitioners use some form of acronym when noting the responses, such as a tick next to DCN and no RAPD. Others write PERRL (representing pupils equal, round and respond to light and accommodation). With defective pupil responses, a description of the exact defect needs to be recorded.

- Anisocoria which does not respond symmetrically to light may indicate a pathological process such as an efferent defect. Horner's syndrome, for example, will give a unilateral miosis. In the case of a pupil defect or pathological anisocoria (in the absence of any knowledge of the cause already having been established), referral is usually appropriate.

6
Gross perimetry and confrontation

The investigation of visual field is an essential component of any eye examination as it may detect both early ocular and neurological disease processes which other investigations may miss. Detailed and accurate field screening or investigation is a subject covered in depth in a sister book in this series (*Visual Fields* by Robert Cubbidge). Such detailed examinations, though essential, are often not included as part of the basic routine examination and are instead considered supplementary tests. However, because of the significance of the presence of any previously undetected major field loss, a routine should include at least one gross assessment of the visual field as any major defect not only emphasizes the need for a more detailed field assessment, but may change the priority of other tests. A large and previously undetected hemianopia should make the practitioner consider referral rather than spending unnecessary time on subjective refraction, for example. It might also be argued that in many cases this gross assessment is the only assessment of the peripheral field that is to be carried out, most modern screeners assessing only the central 25 to 30 degrees. Though it is true that around 85 percent of field defects fall within this space, the remaining minority affecting the intermediate and far periphery are often greatly clinically significant.

Such defects might result from retinal damage, as with for example chorioretinitis, retinal detachment, a neoplasm or early retinitis pigmentosa. It is also important to remember that many defects due to damage to the visual pathway may also start in the far periphery and only extend into the central field at a later stage. An example might be the superior bitemporal loss due to compression of the chiasma from below by a pituitary adenoma.

Confrontation

Though the terms confrontation and gross perimetry are often used as synonyms, strictly speaking confrontation describes one of several "comparison" tests whereas gross perimetry is the use of a target to measure the extent of the visual field and to map any large scotomas within the field. One form of confrontation involves the use of a target moved along an imaginary flat plane between and perpendicular to the gaze of the patient and the practitioner. This obviously will not allow the temporal extent of field to be measured, but will allow the practitioner to confirm that any areas they see can also be seen by the patient. One could also describe other tests as confrontation tests, for example, the presentation of two red targets to the hemifields of the patient to find out whether one of the targets is desaturated, or the use of a shiny coin in four quadrants of the field of one eye. Many confrontation tests are used by neurologists in investigating possible neurological lesions.

One interesting phenomenon, sometimes seen in a partial or relative hemianopia, is where a target is seen on the affected side but disappears when a second target is presented in the adjacent hemifield. This so-called extinction phenomenon gives useful yet quickly and simply obtained information regarding the depth of the hemianopia. Most practitioners use gross fields assessment to measure the extent of the visual field and instead use a form of gross perimetry.

Gross perimetry

Gross perimetry describes the use of a hand-held target held at a constant distance from the patient's eye which, when brought in an arc from beyond their visual field boundary, allows them to announce when the target is first seen (the extent of field or boundary for that particular target size and color). When the target is moved further within their field to the central point of fixation it allows any large defect to be detected.

The choice of target dictates the extent of the isopter, just as with any kinetic assessment. A larger target will be seen at a greater eccentricity, while the isopter for a small target will be contracted. Similarly, a white target brought from beyond the field will be seen before a red target which will itself be

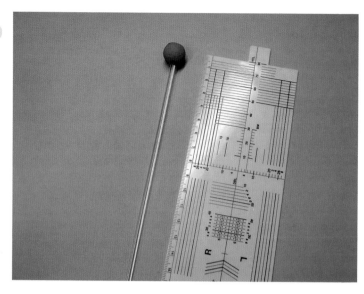

Figure 6.1 A 15 mm diameter red target may be used

seen before a green target. In practice, though a small white target might be justifiable in terms of sensitivity, a red target is generally chosen as it will contrast better with typical wall coverings within the consulting room. To maintain some degree of correlation with a 5 mm white target (typical for gross perimetry), a 15 mm diameter red target may be used instead, its extra size counteracting the reduced sensitivity to red compared to white (Figure 6.1).

The extent of the absolute visual field is dependent upon the shape of the head of the patient, but it is important to remember that the extent of the temporal field is almost always greater than 90 degrees. Typical values are 100 degrees temporally, 75 degrees inferiorly, and 60 degrees nasally and superiorly. The last two are most patient-dependent because of variable nose and brow size. To ensure a starting point beyond the visual field of the patient, therefore, the target should be held somewhat behind them for the temporal measurement.

Method

- As far as is possible in a cluttered consulting room, the surroundings should be as uniform and regular in color and contrast as is practicable.
- The patient should face the practitioner and occlude one eye. No correction should be worn by the patient. Though their hand may be used, this is not fully reliable as many people cannot resist the urge to peek through small gaps between the fingers. An alternative would be for them to be given an occluder and helped to maintain this in front of one eye such that the field of that eye is effectively excluded (Figure 6.2).
- Fixation shifts are one of the main causes of error in any field assessment technique and gross perimetry is no exception.

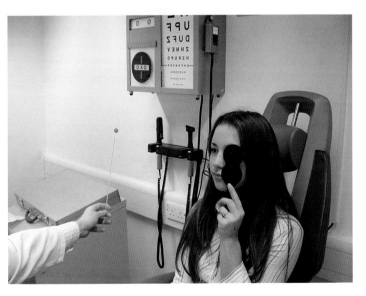

Figure 6.2 Give the patient an occluder to maintain in front of one eye such that the field of that eye is effectively excluded

The patient should be directed to stare with their uncovered eye either at the bridge of the nose or into one of the practitioner's eyes and the practitioner should monitor a steady fixation throughout the test.

- The target should be held at about 35 cm from the patient's eye and initially outside the field of view of the patient.
  The patient should then be told to say when they are first aware of the target as it is slowly but steadily moved around the imaginary arc (always at a constant distance from the eye). Once this position is reached (and a mental note made of it), the target should continue its passage to the center of the patient's view and the patient asked to report any point at which it disappears. If such is reported, the target may be moved about in this blind spot to find a rough outline of the area.

- This should be repeated in eight directions (superior, superior temporal, temporal, inferior temporal and so on). The same should then be carried out for the other eye. Though many practitioners speed up the technique and use only the four main meridians, this may result in a large quadrantanopia being missed.

- The most common error introduced in this method is the failure to maintain a constant distance from the patient's eye. The closer the target is to the eye, the less sensitive the test as a small target movement will subtend a larger area of retina. Only very gross defects will be detected (so the assessment will have a high specificity). The further from the eye the target is, the more sensitive the test but the more difficult the target will be to spot for those without any defect (so specificity will reduce). 35 cm is useful as it is usually comfortable for the practitioner, roughly equates to a bowl perimeter such as the Goldmann or the Humphrey VFA, and offers a reasonable balance of specificity and sensitivity (though both are not particularly high values due to the very gross nature of the test).

- Assuming the isopters equate roughly to typical values for the absolute visual field and there are no major defects within the field, the result should be noted as full on the record card. There are many perfectly innocuous situations where the field may be contracted, for example, the restricted superior field of an elderly patient due to ptosis. This should be noted on the record as such and not ignored.

7
Objective refraction

Introduction

Objective refraction includes retinoscopy or the use of autorefractors, which are appearing in optometric practice in increasing numbers. In general, objective methods are not required to give us a final prescription. They merely need to get us to a point from which subjective methods can take us to the end point accurately and quickly. With an alert and compliant subject it is possible to get an accurate result using subjective methods alone, but it takes time. In general, excessively prolonged refraction of normal patients is usually indicative of poor technique rather than "professionalism". With practice, and if a previous prescription is known, objective refraction should take seconds rather than minutes.

There are patients who are unable to participate in a subjective refraction, because of limitations of understanding or communication. The very young, those with Alzheimer's disease or a learning disability may require that a prescription is arrived at purely from the objective findings. We should have realistic expectations of retinoscopy. It seems that there is only a 50 percent probability that two consecutive measurements of sphere power would be within 0.40D. Cylinder axis is the most repeatable, followed by cylinder power, then sphere power. And unless you are fully ambidextrous you are likely to be better with one eye than the other. Of course, the skill of the examiner will influence both accuracy and repeatability.

Measuring pupillary distance

It is important that we set up the trial frame accurately, because failure to do so may introduce significant artifacts into the final result. Use a frame rule and instruct the patient to look first at your left eye. Line up the zero cursor with the temporal limbus. The patient now looks at your right eye, and the position of the nasal limbus is measured, ensuring that you have not moved the rule meanwhile.

The pupillary distance for near may be measured by instructing the patient to look at the bridge of your nose. The zero is lined up using the left eye and the PD read using the right eye as before. Quite why you would wish to do this is another matter. The actual amount of inset required will vary with both the PD and working distance of the patient, so unless you know these and place your nose in precisely the right position, the measurement is of dubious value. The actual inset required is shown in Table 7.1.

Adjusting the trial frame

The optical centers of the trial frame should be set to the distance PD. If there is marked facial asymmetry you may need to measure monocular PDs and adjust the trial frame accordingly. Later, when you move on to near vision tests the optical centers can be adjusted to equal the near PD, and dropped slightly by adjusting the nosepiece of the trial frame. However, this should only be done if the spectacles that you intend to prescribe are to be set for near vision only. On a pre-presbyopic patient the optical centers should stay set for distance throughout the refraction, as the near ocular motor balance will be affected by the centration of the lenses (Table 7.1).

Table 7.1 **Binocular inset appropriate for specific PDs**

PD	Binocular inset for near vision at:	
	33 cm	40 cm
74 mm	5.5 mm	4.5 mm
70 mm	5.0 mm	4.5 mm
66 mm	5.0 mm	4.0 mm
62 mm	4.5 mm	4.0 mm
58 mm	4.5 mm	3.5 mm
56 mm	4.0 mm	3.5 mm

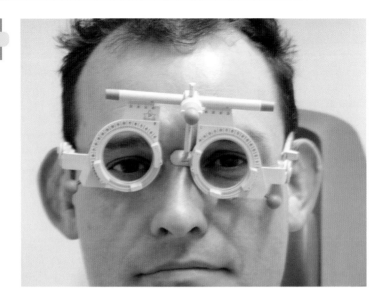

Figure 7.1 Look at the trial frame and check that it is level

- Look at the trial frame and check that it is level, allowing for any facial asymmetries that may be present (Figure 7.1). If the frame is not level, the cylinder axis that you find may be wrong, and vertical prismatic effects may cause artifacts on binocular tests.
- Check that the pantoscopic angle of the frame is sensible (Figure 7.2). If the frame is wrongly tilted, high-powered prescriptions may throw up significant errors in both sphere and cylinder.
- Make sure that the back vertex distance is sensible. If the power of the sphere you find is over ±4.00 DS you should measure the BVD and note it on the final Rx.

Adding lenses to the trial frame

- Place spheres in the back cells of the trial frame. Where you are using more than one sphere in the trial frame the most powerful should be at the back to minimize the effect of

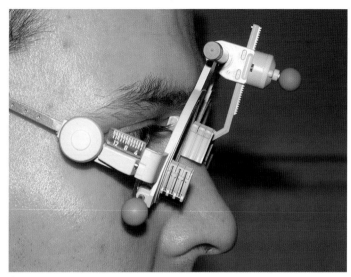

A

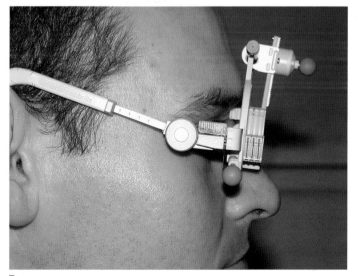

B

Figure 7.2 Check that the pantoscopic angle of the frame is sensible

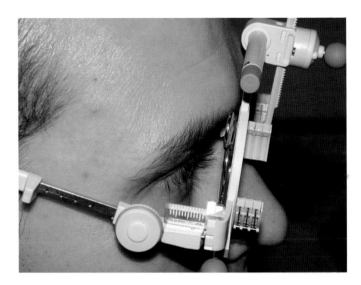

Figure 7.3 The most powerful sphere should be placed in the first of the rear cells

vertex distance. However, if you are using an Oculus™ or similar trial frame, which incorporates a built-in vertex distance scale, the most powerful sphere should be placed in the first of the rear cells (the back cell one nearest the front) (Figure 7.3). This is the cell to which the scale is referenced.

- When you change spheres, try to ensure that the patient is never grossly under-plussed when you change lenses. It is best to add the next plus lens before you remove the current one. It can be tricky with modern trial frames but it becomes easier with practice.
- It is essential to make sure that all lenses are thoroughly clean throughout refraction. Experience suggests this is often not the case.

A note on phoropters

Increasingly, phoropter heads are used instead of trial frames (Figure 7.4). Modern automated lens carriages allow fast lens

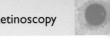

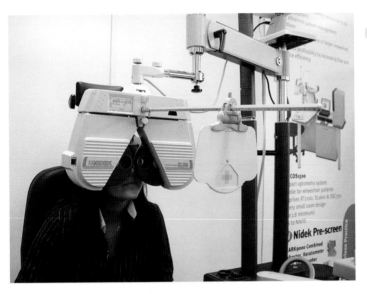

Figure 7.4 Increasingly, phoropter heads are used instead of trial frames

insertion, greater accuracy in axis location, more rapid comparison presentation of lenses, use of variable prism, and a variety of further options depending on the model, such as immediate comparison of new refractive findings with previous results. They are not advisable for a few situations, notably low-vision assessment and over-refraction of multifocal contact lenses, where the reduced light levels may affect visual performance or pupil size respectively and may hinder binocular assessment.

Retinoscopy

Target

Ideally, we want a target that will promote accurate and steady fixation but no stimulus to accommodation. Various targets are used and they probably make little difference to the end result, but there is some evidence that the rings on the green block of the duochrome might be the ones that produce least accommodation. In the absence of any contradictory evidence the rings on the green would be the recommended fixation target for retinoscopy.

Light conditions

A darkened room will cause pupil dilation and make the retinoscope reflex more visible, though complete darkness can stimulate accommodation. It might also be difficult to find the trial lenses.

Position

You must try to work within 5 degrees of the visual axis, both horizontally and vertically. Adjust the chair height for vertical alignment, allowing for the fact that the test chart may be above the patient, so the patient may be looking slightly upward. Errors of the order of $-0.50DC \times 90$ occur if 10 degrees off horizontally. Unless you have reduced vision in one eye use your right eye to test the patient's right eye, and your left eye for the patient's left eye. If this is impossible, the Barratt method should be employed (see page 89). For horizontal alignment, get the patient to look at the green of the duochrome, get your head in the way and ask the patient to tell you when they can just see the green panel. Ask the patient to tell you if your head gets in the way.

Working distance

You should work at a distance that allows you to change the lenses in the trial frame without changing body position, and for most people this means that the working distance will be less than the 2/3 m which seems to be the expected norm. Only the tall can reach if they work at 2/3 m and for many 1/2 m is more realistic. It doesn't matter what the distance is provided you know how much to allow for your working lens and the distance is maintained throughout the test. Measure your customary working distance so that you know how much spherical power

Table 7.2 Appropriate lens allowance for working distance

Working distance (cm)	Working lens allowance (D)
50	2.00
57	1.75
66	1.50
80	1.25
100	1.00

to allow for it. Make sure that you can return to it by measuring with your arm. Usually the base of the fingers or the wrist is used as a reference point, as this allows you to change lenses without moving your body position. Check your working distance when you have moved from it (e.g. to change a lens). If your working distance allowance is wrong, errors in the power of the sphere (and usually the cylinder too) will result. For example, if you are 100 mm out at 2/3 m the sphere will be approximately 0.25D in error. Note, however, that the shorter the working distance, the greater the error that will be introduced by 100 mm variation (Table 7.2).

Fogging

During retinoscopy, it is the fixating eye that controls accommodation, so it must be fogged to ensure that accommodation is relaxed. However, if you overdo it, you can induce accommodation, so the fogging should be less than 2.00D.

Initially both eyes should be corrected with what you think is likely to be the full plus correction, based on the patient's existing correction (if available), VA, and symptoms and history, plus the working distance allowance. Check with the retinoscope that you have an "against" movement in either eye. From time to time during retinoscopy, pass the retinoscope beam across the fixating eye to make sure that it is still fogged. This is particularly important with young hyperopic patients.

Initial lens

If you have the patient's last spectacle prescription, this is a good starting point. If the patient has lost their spectacles and no previous prescription is available, consider the unaided vision and far point. A little thought at this stage can save a lot of time and effort. There is nothing to stop you checking the VA when you have neutralized the more positive meridian, to get an idea of the cylinder power required.

Distance unaided vision is related to refractive error in myopes and manifest hyperopes (Table 7.3).

In purely astigmatic refractive errors (or with the best vision sphere in place (Table 7.4)):

- It is important to remember that these are only average values. Patients with small pupils (usually presbyopes) will experience less blur per diopter, and those with large pupils more. For myopes, the far point at which small print can be seen clearly varies inversely with refractive error (Table 7.5).
- The working lens should be incorporated into the correcting sphere. The use of a separate working lens introduces an extra set of reflections and uses up one of the trial frame spaces you may need for the patient's prescription. For the ideal starting point, we would want the patient **slightly** fogged (overplussed)

Table 7.3 **Expected vision for any uncorrected mean sphere**

Vision	Equivalent sphere (myopia/manifest hyperopia)
6/5	Plano
6/6	0.25–0.50 DS
6/9	0.50–0.75 DS
6/12	0.75–1.00 DS
6/18	1.00–1.25 DS
6/24	1.25–1.75 DS
6/36	1.75–2.25 DS

Table 7.4 Expected vision for any uncorrected cylinder

Vision	Equivalent cylinder (with best vision sphere in place)
6/9	1.00–1.25 DC
6/12	1.25–1.75 DC
6/18	1.75–2.25 DC
6/24	2.50–3.00 DC
6/36	3.00–4.00 DC

for distance to discourage accommodation, but rather less than 2.00D. The easiest type of reflex to interpret is a quick "with" movement which should occur if the patient is slightly underplussed for your working distance. They will still be somewhat fogged for the distance that the patient is fixating as your retinoscope and the patient are separated by 1.50D.

Plus or minus cylinder?

Plus cylinders do tend to give a clearer, more easily neutralized streak and are favored by some practitioners who rely on retinoscopy to provide a final prescription (e.g. working with special needs patients). However, using minus cylinders does

Table 7.5 Variation of far point with uncorrected myopia

Spherical refractive error (diopters)	Far point (cm)
2.00	50
4.00	25
6.00	16.7
8.00	12.5
10.00	10
12.00	8.3

ensure that accommodation is better controlled and most automated refractor heads do not have a plus-cylinder option. Minus-cylinders are more commonly used in routine refraction.

Streak or spot?

Either type of retinoscope will do the job, in the hands of someone familiar with it. Streak retinoscopes are currently fashionable and they do make axis determination easier where there are high cylinders, but spot retinoscopes probably make it easier to deal with lower levels of astigmatism. Some retinoscopes now come with a choice of bulb, so practitioners can experiment for themselves.

Streak retinoscopy

Initially the retinoscope should be set to give maximum divergence (the collar should be down). The beam is swept along the 90° and 180° meridians and the reflex observed. If the patient's principal meridians lie along 90° and 180° the reflex within the pupil will be seen to move parallel to the direction that you are sweeping. If not, the reflex moves obliquely to the direction of sweep. With medium to high degrees of astigmatism, this deviation is apparent even when the beam is static (Figure 7.5). Rotating the streak will align the reflex and the direction of sweep (Figure 7.6). When the two coincide, you are sweeping along one of the principal meridians, the other being at 90° if the astigmatism is regular.

Neutralize the more positive or least negative meridian first. To decide which this is:

- If you have a "with" movement in both meridians, the meridian showing the slowest movement is the more positive.
- If you have "with" in one meridian and "against" in the other, the meridian showing the "with" movement is the more positive.
- If you have an "against" movement in both meridians, that showing the faster movement is the more positive or least negative.

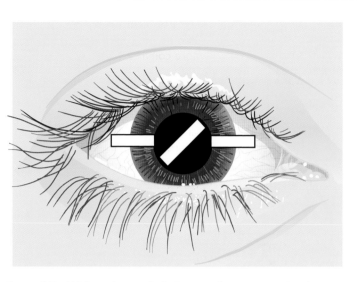

Figure 7.5 With medium to high degrees of astigmatism, this deviation is apparent even when the beam is static

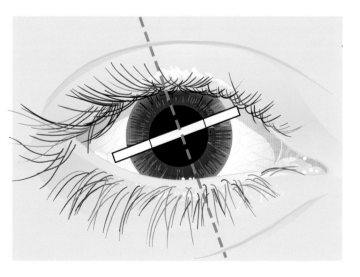

Figure 7.6 Rotating the streak will align the reflex and the direction of sweep

When you think you have reversal, use a **bracketing** technique to check.

For power
- Move slightly backwards and forwards. The reflex should change from "against" to "with".
- Use ±0.25D twirls. Again the reflex should change from "against" to "with".

For axis (Lindner's method)
- Neutralize the more positive meridian.
- Sweep the beam across meridians at +45° and –45° to the axis of the trial cylinder. The reflexes should be identical. If one is "with" and one "against", move the axis toward the meridian showing "with" movement.

Small cylinders
If small cylinders are present, either:

1. Move the collar up.
- Neutralize the more positive meridian.
- Move the collar up so that the immediate source is between the retinoscope and the eye. You should see a narrow reflex which moves rapidly in a **reversed** direction. Therefore a "with" movement is seen, which is neutralized with negative lenses. This technique is also useful as a check test, and in high ametropia where no initial reflex can be seen.

2. Use the Francis method.
- Neutralize the more positive meridian.
- Set the collar for maximum divergence (i.e. down). The immediate source will lie behind the retinoscope at about 1 m with a working distance of 2/3 m.
- Add –0.50DS. The reflex will become a narrow line.
- Rotate the beam through 90°. If the reflex stays narrow, no significant astigmatism is present. Even a tiny amount

causes the reflex to fill the pupil as the beam completes its rotation. The orientation of the beam that produces the narrowest reflex is 90° off the minus cylinder axis.
- Add +0.50DS and neutralize the second meridian.

Alternative methods

There are a number of methods that may be worth trying if conventional methods are not possible or are not working on a particular patient.

Parker method
- Identify the meridians in the usual way.
- Set the streak along the axis, and adjust the streak to give a minimum width reflex.
- As the ametropia is corrected, the width of the streak increases. When the reflex fills the pupil the ametropia is neutralized.

Barratt method
The patient fixates a bright luminous fixation object binocularly. The target should ideally be non-accommodative though the retinoscope target often used is not, completely. Alternatively the practitioner's forehead may act as the target.

Advantages claimed include:

- Working closer to the visual axis.
- Smaller pupil due to near reflex. Fewer aberrations as a result (but also a less bright reflex).
- Only one of the practitioner's eyes is used. This makes the method particularly useful for those optometrists with reduced acuity in one eye.

The disadvantage is that the patient will accommodate, especially younger ones. The sphere must be checked with distance fixation in one eye either before or after using the Barratt method and the final result adjusted accordingly.

Near retinoscopy

Mohindra's technique (1975) is a development of near-fixation retinoscopy which allows refraction of infants and young children without the use of cycloplegics. The room lights are slowly extinguished and the child encouraged to look at the retinoscope light. It is usual to ask the parent to occlude one eye, though opinions vary as to whether this makes a significant difference. Feeding tends to relax accommodation. The pupil will initially constrict but after a few seconds dilation will occur. At this point the refractive error may be neutralized. Lens racks may be used for speed, each meridian being neutralized separately. Accurate fixation may be encouraged in older children by asking the child when they can see "the black spot in the light" (i.e. the sight hole in the mirror, on a spot retinoscope).

The working distance is usually 0.5 m, so the expected allowance for the working distance would be 2.00D. However, near retinoscopy does tend to underestimate hyperopia, so a correction factor of 1.25D is used for adults, though it has been suggested that a correction factor of 1.00D is appropriate for children older than 2 years and 0.75D for those younger.

Opinions vary on the accuracy of this technique, particularly in infants and those with higher refractive errors.

Spot retinoscopy

Spot retinoscopy is performed in the same way as streak retinoscopy but the reflex is circular in a patient without significant astigmatism. An astigmatic patient will give a reflex that is elliptical, and this shape and the movement of the reflex relative to the direction of sweep (which is the same as with a streak) enables rapid identification of the degree and axis of astigmatism. It is usually recommended that the more positive meridian is neutralized before correcting the cylinder, but you may find that it is easier to do when you have a rapid "with" movement in this meridian. This means that you are 0.25D to 0.50D under-plussed for the distance you are working at, but the patient should still be fogged for their fixation distance. The cylinder power is increased until the reflex is circular and its speed in the two principal meridians is the same, then you add the final bit of sphere.

Tips for difficult retinoscopy

Split reflex

This can occur in keratoconus, corneal scarring or lens changes.
Check that the trial lenses are clean, correctly centered and that you
are working on axis. Don't try to obtain reversal, use bracketing.

Opacities

You may have to work around them by moving off axis. Allow for
this when estimating the cylinder. It might also be necessary to
work closer to obtain a brighter reflex.

Ocular abnormalities

Localized bulges or asymmetries may mean that the fovea is on a
different plane to the slightly off-axis point that forms the reflex.
Therefore the sphere power may be some way out.

Accommodative tonus

In young hyperopes the retinoscope result will often be considerably
more positive than the eventual subjective refraction due to high
accommodative tonus. Patience is a virtue here if you suspect
that there might be more plus to add. Keep sweeping the beam
across, keep reminding the patient to look at the circles on the
green, and eventually you will see a "with" movement, albeit a
transient one. Neutralize it, and repeat until you are sure that all of
the hyperopia is corrected. If you are consistently underplussing on
retinoscopy, check your working distance, and slow down.

The stenopaic slit

This is an elongated pinhole which is used to find an approximate
correction of astigmatism in cases where retinoscopy will not give
an accurate result and high astigmatism is suspected. It is placed
before the eye being tested with the BVS in place. The slit is rotated
slowly and the position that gives the patient the best acuity is
noted. This approximates one of the principal meridians of the eye.

- With the slit still in place, + and − spheres are added to give a
  "best vision sphere" for this meridian.

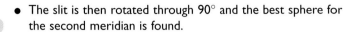

- The slit is then rotated through 90° and the best sphere for the second meridian is found.

The powers found are then converted to sphero-cylindrical form and the result placed in the trial frame, where it can be refined by normal subjective techniques if appropriate. It must be remembered that the axis is at right angles to the power meridian.

Non-refractive uses of retinoscopy

Retinoscopy may be performed before ophthalmoscopy, so it may be the first chance to view the internal structure of the eye. A number of conditions may alter the appearance of the reflex:

- The light reflected from the retina retroilluminates the lens, iris and cornea. Opacities in the lens and iris can be seen as dark areas against the red background. The same effect may be observed with an ophthalmoscope held about 30–40 cm from the patient's eye. Early opacities may be easier to see by retroillumination than by direct observation with the ophthalmoscope.
- Where extensive transillumination defects are present in uveitis or pigment dispersion syndrome it may be possible to see them as bright radial streaks on the iris. However, the slit lamp is a better instrument to observe this.
- Keratoconus distorts the reflex and produces a swirling motion.
- Retinal detachment involving the central area will distort the reflecting surface and a gray reflex may be seen.
- A tight soft contact lens will have apical clearance in the central area which will cause distortion of the reflex.
- It is possible to perform indirect ophthalmoscopy with a retinoscope and a high plus lens, provided the instrument is bright enough.

Autorefractors

The use of a machine to measure refractive error has a long history. The original optometers could use either subjective methods (the forerunners of modern phoropters) or objective methods and it is the automated objective refraction instruments that are now described as autorefractors. Autorefractors use an infrared light source (around 800 to 900 nm) which allows good ocular transmission, but requires a −0.50D adjustment to the final refraction due to error introduced by reflection from the choroid and sclera. The source projects light via a beam splitter and a Badal lens system to form a slit image within the eye, the reflection of which passes out via the beam splitter to reach a light sensor. Throughout, the patient is encouraged to relax accommodation (a major source of error for autorefractor measurement) by use of a fixation target or, in some cases, an open view to allow fixation on a distant target. The calculation of refractive error is based upon analysis of how the patient's eye influences the infrared radiation.

The way this analysis is performed varies. Most of the original instruments used some form of image quality analysis, relying on positioning of the Badal lens system to achieve a maximum signal to the light sensor. The majority of modern autorefractors, of which there are many, rely on an adapted Scheiner disk principle. The original Scheiner disk consisted of two holes in a card placed before the eye. A myopic eye will see the two images from the holes swapped over or crossed, while the hypermetrope sees them uncrossed. This may be done in various meridians to give information about the nature of astigmatism. Autorefractors simulate this using LED light sources, the images of which are detected by a light sensor or photodetector, and the position of the LED needed to achieve a single image over the photodetector is related to the patient refractive error. A further method employed by a few machines is an adaptation of retinoscopy, where the instrument analyzes the speed of movement of a reflex of infrared light to measure the refractive error.

Most studies suggest that autorefractors are quick, simple, repeatable and accurate (with some qualification). With cycloplegia or good accommodative control the results are very accurate. Indeed the spherical aberration introduced by the dilation of a cycloplegic makes the method preferable to retinoscopy in many cases. Its ease of use makes it suitable to be carried out by ancillary staff, so reducing the burden on the optometrist. The machines may directly link to an automated phoropter head, again making the routine refraction more fluid. It is useful to remember that even the most accurate objective measurement may not be that preferred by the patient so a subsequent subjective examination is always preferable to ensure a tolerable refractive error, even though this is sometimes modified away from the actual refractive error present.

The main source of error is due to poor fixation (dependent very much on the target of the instrument), accommodative fluctuation (proximal accommodation in the young invariably leads to overminussed measurements) and media difficulties (which are likely to reduce the effectiveness of retinoscopy also). The lack of portability of the instruments is less of an issue nowadays as several portable models exist, and some have found use in child screening programs (Figure 7.7) where the main outcome is not

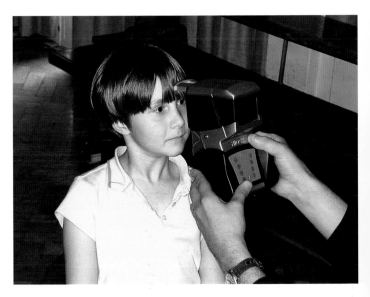

Figure 7.7 Several portable models of autorefractors have found use in child screening programs

precise error measurement but detection of large amounts of ametropia or anisometropia. Other new models incorporate some subjective assessment also, with the patient responding to prompts to clarify a presented image.

Cycloplegic refraction

When should cycloplegic refraction be done?

This is included in this chapter rather than that devoted to subjective refraction on the grounds that most "cyclos" are performed on children whose subjective responses are not entirely reliable. Some practitioners advocate cycloplegic examination of all new child patients. This has the advantage of providing more reliable baseline data on the refractive error at the expense of time and some trauma for the patient.

In general optometric practice, most practitioners tend to use cycloplegics when:

- There is undiagnosed manifest esotropia.
- An esotropia has been noticed by the parent or guardian.
- There is unstable or uncompensated esophoria.
- There are significant risk factors for esotropia and amblyopia (family history, significant refractive error, birth history, etc.).
- A satisfactory level of acuity is not obtained in one or both eyes.
- Stereoscopic acuity is unsatisfactory/absent.
- Latent hyperopia or pseudomyopia is suspected.

Should I use an anesthetic first?

Cycloplegics sting and very few children seem entirely grateful for the experience. This can be ameliorated somewhat by the use of proxymetacaine 0.5 percent, a local anesthetic. This stings rather less than the other local anesthetics used on the eye, and will remove the sting of the subsequent cycloplegic entirely. A further advantage is that the absorption of the cycloplegic will be enhanced. Proxymetacaine is available in minims, but it needs to be stored in the fridge, which is not possible at all practices.

The only other drawback would be if the patient did not like the first drop, and decided to resist the instillation of the second.

Which cycloplegic?

At one time it was common practice to hand out atropine sulfate to the patient's parents to administer at home for three days prior to the examination. In these less innocent times, this potentially fatal hallucinogen has become rather less popular in the high street and patients requiring it would normally be referred to a specialist clinic.

Cyclopentolate is the most popular cycloplegic agent. The 1 percent solution is suitable for most patients. One drop is usually enough, but for patients with dark iridies a second drop may be needed if nothing seems to be happening after 15 minutes. It does not produce absolute cycloplegia, but the residual accommodative tonus is less than 1.50 diopters. No "tonus allowance" needs to be made, so you can prescribe the "full cyclo" if you need to (and only if). The 0.5 percent solution is needed for children under 3 months, though few would be encountered in the general ophthalmic services.

Tropicamide 1 percent has been found to be a useful, if short-acting, cycloplegic for patients in their late teens and older. In adult patients, the short duration is a virtue and this is the ideal agent to investigate the adult patient who you think might be a latent hyperope or a pseudomyope. Two drops, approximately 5 minutes apart following proxymetacaine, is generally recommended.

See Table 7.6 for a comparison of atropine, cyclopentolate and tropicamide.

How do I get the drops in?

Children are rarely tremendously keen on having drops put in.

- Explain what you are going to do in a calm way. Avoid words like "sting" and "pain". Tell the patient that the drops "might feel a bit funny". Try to avoid lying to the child.
- Watch your body language, as children are rather good at reading it. You need to be sending out the signals that reinforce your spoken advice.

Table 7.6 **Comparison of atropine, cyclopentolate and tropicamide**

Agent	Onset of adequate cycloplegia	Duration of cycloplegia	Duration of mydriasis	Tonus allowance needed?
Atropine	36 hours	7–10 days	10–14 days	Yes (?)
Cyclopentolate	30–60 minutes	Up to 12 hours	24–48 hours	No
Tropicamide	30 minutes	2–6 hours	8–9 hours	No

- Sitting on mother's lap is a safe place to be for most small children.
- The child might move fairly suddenly, and you don't want to stick a minim in their eye. If they are cooperating, get the patient to look down, raise the upper lid gently with your thumb and keep the neck of the minim against the thumb while you instill the drop. If the patient moves, so does your thumb and so will the minim.
- If the child will not open their eyes a variation of an old contact lens trick can be useful. While trying to raise the upper lid with your thumb, out of the blue say "Now, open your mouth as wide as you can!" It's almost impossible to open your mouth wide and close your eyes tight at the same time.
- If the child closes their eyelids and steadfastly refuses to open them, three drops on the upper lashes at the lid margin will generally ensure some drops enter the eye.

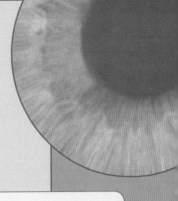

8
Subjective refraction

Introduction

With retinoscopy completed the examiner can proceed to the subjective stage of refraction. In an ideal world, what you now have in the trial frame is the patient's full spectacle correction plus your working lens. The accurate correction of the astigmatic error requires that the circle of least confusion (CLC) is placed on the retina and kept there while the cross-cylinder is in use. If this is not achieved, both the axis and power found will be wrong. The range of spherical powers that allow maximum acuity can be several diopters in patients with small pupils and low acuities, though it is usually smaller. There may be a unique value for the correction which gives maximum contrast, though where accommodation is active this may also be a range. In this latter case the most positive lens that gives maximum contrast is usually the optimum correction.

The recommended routine includes a rather elaborate sequence of checks on the sphere power before, during and after the cross-cylinder is used. This is to ensure that:

- The patient has not been under-plussed. This is particularly easy with young patients, especially hyperopes.
- The initial sphere will be within the effective range of the duochrome test.

Binocular versus monocular refraction

It seems remarkable that more students of optometry enter their pre-registration year performing monocular refractions than binocular ones. Some university clinics appear to take the view that monocular refraction is easier to learn, which seems a little patronizing when applied to honors degree students. Binocular refraction has no major disadvantages when compared to monocular refraction, though there are patients who cannot be refracted binocularly.

Advantages of binocular refraction

- Accommodation is suspended with a plus sphere, and tied to convergence.
- No separate binocular balancing is needed. This saves quite a lot of time.
- Where latent nystagmus is present, it will be reduced.
- Rotational phorias (cyclophorias), if present, will not reduce the final binocular VA. This is now known to be an important factor in refractive surgery patients, and binocular refraction is required in the clinical protocols for pre-treatment refractions in some refractive surgery clinics.

Limitations

Binocular refraction should not be used where acuities are markedly unequal, or one eye is strongly "dominant". If you do start to apply it to an unsuitable patient, they will usually tell you fairly quickly ("Should I be seeing double?"). In such cases occlude the better eye, refract the worst eye. Then refract the better eye with the worst eye fogged, if necessary, or even unfogged if the acuity is considerably worse than the eye you are going to test. If the worst eye is 6/9 or less, it may be unnecessary to fog it. If the difference is less it is often possible to refract binocularly, but the final decision has to be taken on an individual case basis.

Humphriss immediate contrast (HIC) technique

This method employs a fogging lens before the eye that is not being refracted. Humphriss recommended a +0.75DS lens, though most practitioners use a +1.00DS and some have used their retinoscope working lens (i.e. +1.50DS) and claim it works as well. The idea is to reduce the acuity in this eye to about 6/12, at which point central vision is inhibited and the "physiological septum" is established. The first eye is then refracted. When the end point is reached, the eye that was fogged is occluded, and the eye that was refracted is fogged by +1.00DS. Provided that the +1.00DS blur test reduces the acuity to a satisfactory level, it can be left in as the fogging lens while the second eye is refracted. If the +1.00DS does not reduce the acuity enough, add more plus until it does.

The "Hack Humphriss" technique

This is one of those terribly useful and commonly employed techniques that never seem to find their way into the textbooks. However, it works so well that many practitioners use it as their basic technique. Essentially, this is a mixture between binocular and monocular refraction.

- To refract the right eye, occlude the left eye.
- Refract the right eye monocularly.
- Apply the +1.00DS blur test. If the VA is reduced to 6/12 or so leave the +1.00DS in. If not, adjust the fogging lens until it does.
- Refract the left eye with the right eye fogged, i.e. binocularly.
- Apply the +1.00DS blur test to the left eye.
- Check the final sphere balance of the right eye binocularly with the +1.00DS still in place before the left eye.

If you need to add a substantial amount of plus because your retinoscopy result was some way out, it is worth checking the fogged eye periodically to ensure that it is still fogged. Sometimes the addition of plus to the eye being refracted will cause both eyes to relax accommodation.

To place the CLC near the retina

Initially, we must determine the "best vision sphere" (BVS), which can be defined as the most plus or least minus lens with which the patient can enjoy maximum visual acuity. In order that we do not underplus, a "fogging" technique is used. For each eye:

- Check the visual acuities with the working distance lenses still in place. The visual acuity should be approximately 6/24 for a working distance of 66 cm and a working lens of +1.50DS.

If the pupils are small the acuity may be considerably better than this.

- Reduce the plus to give 6/18. At this point you should be about +1.00DS overcorrected.
- Reduce the plus until the VA stops improving (as opposed to going smaller and darker).

To refine the best vision sphere

The sphere may be refined by use of the duochrome or ± spherical twirls. The two methods give statistically identical results, though this does not mean that they will always agree on a particular patient. Using one method to validate the other is generally a waste of time. Each method has some limitations and the techniques must be applied correctly. It is important that you are in control of the patient's accommodation and don't stimulate it unnecessarily. Change plus lenses by inserting the replacement before removing the original, change minus lenses by removing the original before inserting the replacement. This goes for cylinders as well as spheres.

Duochrome

- If the error is over 1.00DS, or the vision 6/9 or worse, the results may be unreliable. The red and green only have a 0.50DS difference in focus.
- Over 55 years of age, the chromatic aberration of the eye drops markedly, so the dioptric interval of the red and green reduces, especially with a small pupil.
- Yellowing of the lens causes a red shift, leading to underplussing.
- It is important that the patient understands that they must compare the **rings** on the duochrome rather than the colors themselves. Some patients concentrate more on the brightness of the rings, others on the basis of favorite colors.
- If the rings on the green are clearer the answer is unambiguous regardless of the patient's age. If they are clearer on the red,

the patient may be myopic or they might be accommodating. To avoid overdoing the minus, patients who see the rings on the red as clearer more often than seems right should also be checked with the other methods below.

Simultan technique (using ±twirls)

- The +lens must be presented **first** for **at least 1 second** to relax accommodation.
- The −lens should not be held for more than **1 second**, which is the reaction time plus response time for accommodation.

The patient is asked "Is it clearer with the first lens, the second lens…or are they both the same?" It is useful to split the two halves of this question to avoid asking a multiple question. The initial comparison should be between more plus and more minus. The third option should only be offered if the patient cannot differentiate between the first two.

If the first lens is clearer or they are both the same, add +0.25. If the second lens is clearer (as opposed to just smaller and darker), add −0.25 to the eye being tested.

The rapidity with which the − lens must be withdrawn can cause problems when a patient is slow to react. For this reason many practitioners have modified the simultan technique to eliminate this phase.

Adding plus only

After initially determining that the sphere is a little (not more than 0.50DS) underplussed by duochrome or simultan, +0.25 is introduced and the question asked: "Is it clearer with the lens, without it…or just the same?" OR "Is it just the same with the lens, or worse?"

The first variant has the disadvantage of being a multiple question. The second may confuse because the +0.25 often is clearer (especially in presbyopes). You must, as always, pick the question to suit the current patient and it is sometimes necessary to change the question once you have got used to the patient.

If in doubt, try both variations in succession and see which one the patient responds to best. If the patient finds the vision clearer or identical with the plus, add +0.25 to the sphere and repeat. If the patient rejects the plus, add −0.25 to the sphere in the trial frame, then repeat.

With this method accommodation may be induced when we add minus power to the sphere in the trial frame, but we are always adding plus, and therefore relaxing accommodation, immediately before the comparison is made.

Placing the CLC on the retina

If the human visual system had no depth of focus, we could use the best vision sphere as it is and proceed to investigate cylindrical power. However, there is a measurable depth of focus even in young patients with big pupils. On older patients with smaller pupils, and on the very astigmatic, whose principal foci will be widely separated, this depth of focus will be larger. Theoretically, the best way to ensure that the CLC is placed precisely on the retina is to allow the patient to put it there with accommodation, assuming they have any. There is actually no real scientific proof that patients do this, and the total amount of blur is higher at the CLC than at other points, but proceeding on this assumption seems to work. We aim therefore to allow the patient to accommodate **minimally** by slightly underplussing them.

For patients who are likely to have a small depth of focus (young patients with low degrees of astigmatism) modifying the BVS by −0.25 is appropriate. For patients with higher degrees of astigmatism or larger depths of focus a larger initial modification may be required.

Cross-cylinder technique

The cross-cylinder is a lens that has a positive cylinder worked on one surface and a numerically equal negative cylinder on the

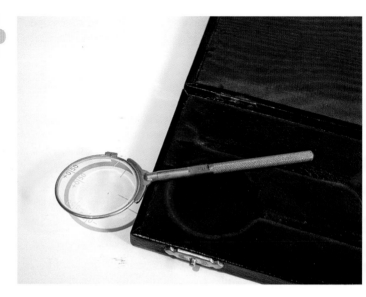

Figure 8.1 The cross-cylinder is a lens that has a positive cylinder worked on one surface and a numerically equal negative cylinder on the other

other (Figure 8.1). The axes of the two cylinders are at right angles to each other. Thus the actual power of a ±0.25 cross-cylinder is equivalent to a spherocylindrical lens of +0.25D spherical and −0.50D cylindrical power. In general, the axes are marked with + and − signs, and usually the plus axis is marked in red and the minus axis in white.

Once you have refined the sphere, there is nothing to stop you checking the VA, as this might indicate how much cylinder remains to be corrected. In general, you will probably have close to the right correction (the "working cylinder") in place, but where the astigmatic error appears small on retinoscopy, it may save time to leave out the cylinder entirely and check initially with a cross-cylinder of a power roughly equal to the estimated astigmatic error over a purely spherical correction. Once the working cylinder has been established it can be refined as follows.

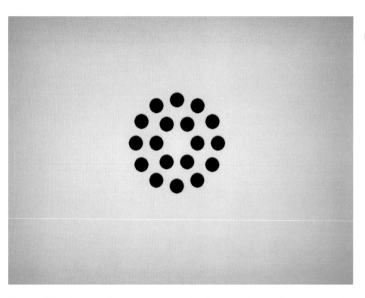

Figure 8.2 Targets for crosscyl examination are chosen based on acuity and tend to be circular

What should the patient look at?

Generally the target should be circular and a little bigger than the smallest letters that can be seen (Figure 8.2), as targets containing linear elements may prejudice the result if the circle of least confusion is not quite on the retina. Some practitioners have advocated using several letters at a time, but this can confuse the patient (not to mention the practitioner) when "some letters are better with position one, and some with position two". Circles or Landolt Cs of the appropriate size, or targets consisting of a pattern of dots, are preferable to single letters (other than Os).

Axis

- The cross-cylinder is presented so that its plus and minus axes lie at 45° to the axis of the working cylinder.

- The cross-cylinder should be presented for at least 1 second in each meridian, and spun as quickly as possible between meridians. Some cross-cylinders have flat areas on the handle to assist this.
- Initially a cross-cylinder of similar or slightly less power than the estimated required cylinder power is ideal. The axis is further refined after determining the power. For large errors of axis a ±0.50 gives a larger difference in image. As the error gets smaller, the ±0.25 gives similar differences but the overall blur and distortion are smaller and less distracting.

Power

- In this case the axes of the cross-cylinder are aligned with that of the working cylinder.
- To check the result, use a bracketing technique by using the cross-cylinder on lenses which are + and −0.25DC from your end point.
- **Remember to modify the sphere when you change the power of the cylinder** in order to keep the circle of least confusion on the retina. As a general rule, every cylinder change should be matched with a change of sphere by half the amount and with the opposite sign (for each −0.50DC, change the sphere +0.25DS). Alternatively, you can check with the duochrome or sphere twirls at intervals. Automated refractor heads modify the sphere automatically. However, if you use one of these in practice, you will probably still be using a trial frame in your final exams. Trial frames rarely remember to change the sphere for you, so that will be your job.

Final axis determination

Recheck the axis with a ±0.25 cross-cylinder. Bracket the end point by checking at 5 degrees either side of the axis found.

What if the patient can't make up their mind?

This may be because they don't understand what they are supposed to be doing. This may be because your instructions are not very explicit, or simply because they can't hear you. Repeat the instructions slowly and clearly. If they can both hear and understand you it may be because the cross-cylinder you are using is of insufficient power to make a discernible difference to the target.

What if the patient always says position one is clearer?

Perseveration can be defined as a tendency of organismic activity to recur without apparent associative stimulus. This is the one-track mind the patient who keeps telling you that the first lens is clearer when you know it can't be, and sometimes even when you ask them a completely different question. Perseverators may also give lower scores on some stereotests due to their inability to adapt.

To counteract perseveration the following strategies may be useful:

- Try to arrange it that the answer to any subjective test that you do is not the same too many times in succession. The use of bracketing techniques is beneficial.
- In some cases, vary the question or the way you phrase it, i.e. "Is it clearer with three or four/five or six/seven or eight?"
- A contrived interruption, such as dropping a pen, may break the sequence. A regular rhythm of question and answer, while often useful with other patients, may only reinforce perseveration.

Fan and block technique

Most, though not all, test charts have a fan and block at the top. It is a useful test to have, especially for those patients who do not respond well to a cross-cylinder. It may actually control accommodation better than the cross-cylinder technique as a fogging technique is employed. However, it is thought to be less accurate than the cross-cylinder technique for small astigmatic errors, and it is a monocular method. The starting point is the best vision sphere, as with cross-cylinder, but then the two techniques diverge. A typical technique is described below:

- Occlude the left eye (usually the right eye is tested first, but for no particular reason).
- Remove the cylinder from the right eye.
- Check the visual acuity.
- Add plus until this drops by one line and the circles on the duochrome are clearer on the red.
- The patient then looks at the fan and is asked to report which line(s) are clearest. Initial selection can be aided by asking "If this was a clock face, what time would the clearest line be pointing to?" The clearest line, or the center line of a group of clear lines, indicates the negative cylinder axis.
- The axis can be refined by using the arrowhead. Rotate the arrow until it points toward the chosen clearest line and adjust the axis until the two arms of the arrowhead appear equally clear/blurred.
- At this stage one of the blocks should be clear, while the other one, which has lines at right angles to the clear one, will be blurred. Add negative cylinder until both blocks are equally clear.
- If all of the lines in the fan seem equally clear to the patient, increase the fogging lens by a further +0.50D and check again. If the lines are still all equally clear, no significant astigmatism is present.
- Reduce the fogging lens to find the best sphere, then repeat for the left eye.

Final sphere check

- If your spherical power was correct when using the cross-cylinder, the patient should be slightly underplussed.

Therefore there is no logical reason to offer more minus to the patient. If the patient needs more minus at this stage, your cross-cylinder has probably got the cylinder wrong, so you would need to check it again.

- If using the duochrome pre-presbyopes are often best left on the green, presbyopes on the red, but there are exceptions. If in doubt, balance equally.
- Young myopes are often used to being slightly overcorrected, and young hyperopes undercorrected.
- Exophores may be happier on the green, as accommodative convergence may help to compensate their phoria. Esophores may be better with more plus.
- Use a +1.00 blur test. With the other eye occluded, the VA should be 6/12 or 6/18, with an average pupil. If it is, you have the physiological septum in place for the other eye if you wish to check the sphere balance binocularly. If it is better, the patient is probably underplussed, unless they have small pupils.

The above points are valid for a 6 m chart. In practice, you may come across projection charts that present an image at 3 m, or at infinity. When working with infinity charts you need no adjustment of the sphere for the testing distance. Direct 6 m charts should in theory cause overplussing of 0.167D, which is why pre-presbyopes like to be left on the green. Presbyopes usually have smaller pupils, giving greater tolerance to blur, and appreciate the slight boost to their mid-distance vision that the extra quarter-diopter gives. Projection charts with a 3 m distance will cause overplussing of 0.33D, so it is customary to add −0.25DS to the distance portion of the subjective findings before prescribing. In the case of a presbyope, any extra minus on the distance prescription should be offset by adding +0.25DS to the reading addition.

"Binocular balancing"

In older textbooks, methods are described whereby the eyes are fogged and the sphere adjusted to give equal acuities in the two eyes, but this is rather missing the point of it all. Many patients have a "better" eye, and if we artificially equalize the acuities the patient may be uncomfortable. It may only be possible to equalize the two by compromising the acuity of the better eye.

The idea of binocular balancing is to balance the **accommodative effort** in the two eyes by uncovering any extra hyperopia which becomes manifest when the patient is binocular. If the patient has no accommodation there is little point in trying to balance it. Some practitioners have advocated trying to balance the depths of focus of the two eyes, but this seems a little eccentric, given that the depth of focus is largely pupil-dependent.

Various methods have been developed to give each eye a separate target without causing complete dissociation, using either a physical septum placed on the chart or mirror, or polarization.

The actual balancing can be done either using the duochrome, or by finding the most plus lens consistent with best acuity for each eye. Where you have performed a binocular refraction, no separate balancing is required. In those cases where binocular refraction is inappropriate, it is unlikely that any of these techniques will give you any worthwhile information.

If all else fails, if the patient is happy, keep the balance the same as the last correction. A change of balance often requires some adaptation on the part of the patient, so it should not be undertaken casually. Some management of the patient's expectations is also required in such circumstances, to avoid unnecessary retests.

Binocular plus

With the patient fixating binocularly, check if +0.25DS is accepted binocularly. This may be incorporated into your final Rx, but allow for testing distance, binocular balance, etc. Using binocular refraction techniques, it is rarely necessary to add binocular plus, but practitioners who use monocular techniques may benefit from this step.

9
Accommodation and the near addition

Introduction

Once we have established a correction for distance vision we can turn our attention to near vision clinically, patients may be divided into three groups:

1. Pre-presbyopes.
2. Early presbyopes.
3. Late presbyopes.

Pre-presbyopes are those who have enough accommodation and accommodative stamina to focus at near to their satisfaction. In these cases the amplitude of accommodation is measured and the two eyes compared as significant differences between them may indicate pathology. Provided the ocular motor balance for near is compensated, no extra correction needs to be made for near. It should be noted that when testing accommodation, convergence and ocular motor balance, the optical centers of the trial frame should remain at the distance setting.

Early presbyopes no longer have sufficient accommodation to provide adequate near vision unassisted. The age of onset will vary with the level of visual task undertaken and with the fixation that it needs to be undertaken at. In other words, if the print is big and bold and you only need to look at it for a short time every day, you won't need reading glasses so soon. And if you are 5 ft 0 in. in your socks you will probably need a reading addition some years before a 6 ft 4 in. colleague (longer arms). Myopes who read with their glasses on can cheat a bit by looking obliquely through the lower part of their spectacles. This is easier when deep frames are in fashion. However, myopes who read without spectacles may enfeeble their accommodation and require an earlier near correction. Most patients in this group are between 40 and 55, but some younger patients who have abnormally low accommodative tonus may also be encountered. The near addition required by an early presbyope depends on both the working distance and the accommodation that the patient still has available, so amplitude of accommodation is still usefully measured. However, in real optometric practice, it is rare for a patient who already has a reading addition to have their accommodative amplitude measured unless there are other clinical indications (e.g. a suspected IIId nerve problem). With that in mind, the early presbyopic group might consist of those patients about to have their first reading addition prescribed, and all of those with pre-existing reading additions dealt with as late presbyopes.

Late presbyopes have no accommodation of their own, so their reading addition is largely determined by the working distance required. Depth of focus will remain and those with small pupil diameters may need a lower reading addition than those with wider pupils. Tall people usually need lower additions. However, the ability to resolve fine detail, especially in low-contrast situations, may decline with age and ocular disease. There may be a need to increase the magnification by increasing the addition, though this will incur a shorter working distance and smaller depth of focus. It is unproductive to try to measure the amplitude of accommodation of patients in this (over 55 years) group, so it is rarely attempted.

Amplitude of accommodation

There is a surprising lack of unanimity, among those who have written on the subject, on the precise method used to measure accommodation in a clinical setting. While acknowledging that dynamic retinoscopy can, with practice, give a useful objective measurement of the accommodative abilities of the patient, most people use one of the many variations of the "push-up" method of Donders. The trouble is that no two practitioners seem to agree what this method is. For a start, we need to consider target size since larger print will allow a greater depth of focus. Strictly speaking, accommodation is the ability to retain resolution at closer working distances, so the target used should equate to the distance acuity, yet some authorities recommend using a paragraph of N5 print, which is the equivalent of a distance acuity of 6/15 or so. Even the point of reference for the measurement is in dispute. Should we use the spectacle plane, the bridge of the nose or the lateral canthus, all of which have their advocates? Then there is the dilemma over whether to do a "push-up" or a "push-up and pull-down" technique.

Method

- The RAF rule is usually used (Figure 9.1), though a "budgie stick" and measuring tape are just as good.
- Bring the target slowly toward the patient along the ruler, with the eyes slightly depressed, until it becomes blurred ("push-up").
- The patient is then asked if he can bring the target back into focus. If he can, then continue to move the target toward the patient (until he can no longer regain clear focus) and note the distance in centimeters from the spectacle plane.
- The target is then moved back until the patient can see it clearly, and this distance is also noted ("pull-back" value).

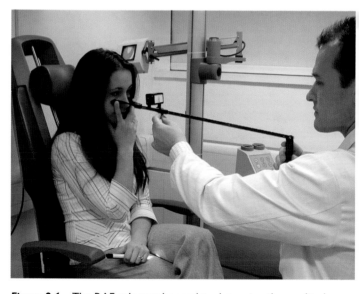

Figure 9.1 The RAF rule may be used to determine the amplitude of accommodation

- The amplitude of accommodation is the average of the "push-up" and "pull-back" values.
- The target should be the smallest print that can be seen clearly when the target is at the remote end of the ruler, or at arm's length if using a budgie stick or separate card.

Accommodation should be measured both monocularly (to screen for IIId nerve anomalies) and binocularly. There are those who advocate repeating each measurement three times to assess the effects of fatigue. There may be value in this approach in some clinical situations, especially in the pediatric area, but in a routine refraction this is rarely a constructive use of time.

Variations of accommodation and reading addition

The normal amplitude of accommodation declines with age until around 55 years, when all that is left is depth of focus. This tends to increase due to the increasing miosis associated with aging (Table 9.1).

Table 9.1 **Expected amplitude of accommodation and reading addition for age**

Age (years)	Expected amplitude (D)	Near addition (DS)
20	10	0
30	8	0
40	5–6	0–0.50
45	3–4	0–1.00
50	2	1.00–1.75
55	(1)	1.50–2.25
60	0	1.75–2.50

There is considerable individual variation in those amplitudes of accommodation that may exist in asymptomatic patients. Reduced accommodation may also be associated with:

- Latent or inadequately corrected hyperopia.
- Poor health (e.g. Graves' disease, alcoholism) or drug treatment (e.g. for asthma, antidepressants) or abuse.
- Hysteria and stress, probably associated with overstimulation of the sympathetic nervous system. Children whose parents have divorced recently, or who are attending a new school, are prone to this.
- Ocular disease (e.g. glaucoma, anterior uveitis, Adie's pupil).
- Myopia. Myopes often read without spectacles and their accommodation may become feeble through disuse. They also tend to have larger pupils, which reduces the depth of focus.
- People who have lived in sunnier climates (e.g. the Gulf) often struggle at near when they come to Britain.
- Students (more usually female) around the age of 12–14 may experience a temporary accommodative palsy which usually resolves spontaneously after a short time. Help with reading may be necessary for a while.

Higher than expected amplitudes of accommodation may be recorded in older patients or those with small pupils due to enhanced depth of focus.

- Patients on pilocarpine will have small pupils and ciliary spasm.
- Some older patients (again more often female) will develop spasm of the near reflex as a response to excessive demands on accommodation or convergence. Often cycloplegia is necessary to rule out myopia.

Starting points for the near addition

- The age of the patient and working distance can be used. Up to 55 years, the following formula may be considered:

Tentative addition = (Age/10) − 3.50D for a working distance of 40 cm

Table 9.2 **Tentative reading additions at increasing range**

Age (years)	Initial addition (DS)
40–45	+0.75–1.00
46–50	+1.25
51–55	+1.50
56–60	+1.75
61–65	+2.00
66–70	+2.25–2.50
70+	+2.50–3.00

After 55, the working distance is the main factor, as accommo-dation has ceased and only depth of focus remains (Table 9.2).

- The correction needed will depend on the accommodation remaining to the patient and their habitual working distance. For early presbyopes both need to be considered. Keep part of the amplitude of accommodation in reserve. Bennett and Francis (1962) suggest leaving one-third of the amplitude of accommodation in reserve. Millodot and Millodot (1989) found that while this was suitable for early presbyopes, an allowance of half of the amplitude was more suitable for women over 52 and men over 63 years.

- The old reading addition, which is what we all really look at in practice, is useful to refer to. Curiously, this is rarely available to undergraduates who are learning to refract, and never to candidates in examinations who are being assessed on their refracting skills. In general, reducing the power (and hence the magnification) should be avoided unless the patient is having problems. Equally, large increases often cause problems with adaptation. The higher the addition, the smaller the depth of focus. The effects of a reduced accommodative stimulus on the ocular motor balance should also be considered ("these new glasses, they draw my eyes").

- Unequal additions are rarely a good idea, unless there are clear reasons (e.g. a unilateral pathological condition affecting ciliary tonus). If you need an unequal addition for no good reason, you probably got the distance sphere balance wrong. Go back and check this first. Occasionally people have been taught to assess and prescribe the addition individually for each eye, but caution must be taken here as the result may reflect differences in depth of focus between the eyes.

Methods of refining the near addition

Given the singular lack of a consensus over the testing of amplitude of accommodation it is probably no surprise that practitioners have found numerous ways to refine the near addition. Whichever is used, the aim is to arrive at an addition (or additions) that will allow clear and comfortable vision at all of the distances at which the patient habitually works. Too little plus, and the patient has to accommodate if they can, or tolerate blur if they cannot. Too much and the depth of focus and ocular motor balance are affected. This would be simple enough if all patients were alike in their tolerance levels to blur, depth of focus and, of course, change in general. Among the more common techniques are the following.

Range of clear vision

This should straddle the most usual reading distance(s) in a way most useful to the patient. Bear in mind any occupational or recreational needs that the patient may have. In some cases it will be impossible to cover all of a patient's requirements with one near addition. Additional pairs may be required to cover part of the range, or multifocals may be required.

Trial lenses

The patient observes a reading card at the preferred reading distance (Figure 9.2). Plus and minus spheres of 0.25D are added

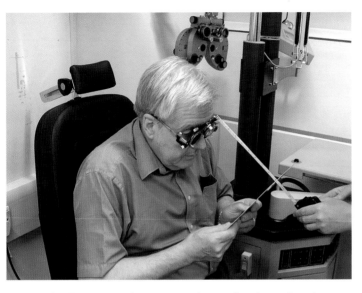

Figure 9.2 The patient observes a reading card at the preferred reading distance

until neither improves the vision. At this point, extra plus will upset the accommodation/convergence relationship, whereas extra minus will require extra accommodative effort.

Near duochrome

Adjust the sphere to give equality or a slight green bias (Figure 9.3). Then check the range by moving nearer and further away. Senile yellowing of the lens causes a red bias and consequent underestimation of positive sphere, but this may not be a bad thing in many cases. Following up with plus and minus trial lenses is a good idea to finalize the result.

Cross-cylinder

A ±0.25D cross-cylinder is placed before the patient's eye monocularly or binocularly with the negative axis at 90°.

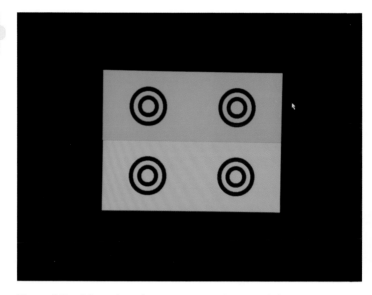

Figure 9.3 Adjust the sphere to give equality or a slight green bias

The patient fixates a grid or cross-target aligned with the axes of the cross-cylinder, placed at their customary working distance. The addition is adjusted to give equal clarity to the vertical and horizontal elements of the target. This is a method often used with automated refractor heads. It is useful to allow the patient to see the target first without the cross-cylinder, then inserting the cross-cylinder and (so that the patient has no time to adjust their accommodation) immediately asking which element of the target is clearer.

Remember, in practice, no one method will be found reliable (if found at all) for all patients and all consulting rooms. Combinations of the above methods and consideration of the patient's needs will generally be the best tactic, so it pays to be familiar with all of these methods.

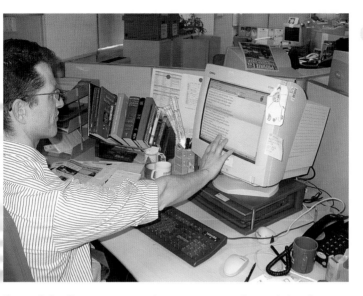

Figure 9.4 Computer terminals are common in the workplace but often a source of visual fatigue

VDU users

The rather archaic term of visual display unit (VDU) is still widely used to describe computer or electronic display screens, now a significant part of most people's visual environment and demands (Figure 9.4).

The Association of Optometrists (AOP) in the UK has issued recommendations on visual standards for VDU users:

1. The ability to read N6 at a distance of 2/3 meter down to 1/3 meter.
2. Monocular vision or GOOD binocular vision. Near phorias over 1/2 prism diopter vertical or 2 prism diopters esophoria and 8 prism diopters exophoria **at working distance** are contraindicated and should be corrected

unless well compensated or deep suppression is present.

3. No central (20 degrees) field defects in the dominant eye.
4. Near point of convergence normal.
5. Clear ocular media checked by **ophthalmoscopy and slit-lamp**.

The above recommendations are intended to increase the level of operator comfort, and therefore efficiency, but failure to achieve the standard does not exclude a person from working with a VDU. Common sense is required when testing VDU users. The recommendations on phoria should not be applied to Maddox rod or wing results, as most people will fail.

10
Extraocular and intraocular examination of the eye

Introduction

There are many techniques employed to visualize both the external eye and adnexa and the internal ocular structures. These are covered in greater detail in a sister book in this series (*Assessment and Investigative Techniques* by Doshi and Harvey).

The Optician's Act does require of any eye examination not just a measurement and correction of the optical status of the eye, but an assessment of the health of the eye and a decision about further management or referral as appropriate. For this reason, any book about the routine examination of the eye must include allusion to this important area.

The exact sequence into which the external and internal examinations fall should be dictated by the particular patient presentation. Someone complaining of a problem with an eyelid or a gritty sensation should obviously be looked at thoroughly on a slit-lamp near the beginning of the assessment. However, in the generic routine taught to undergraduates, slit-lamp examination is usually carried out prior to refraction. Similarly, a myope complaining of flashing lights and visual disturbance warrants ophthalmoscopy almost immediately as immediate referral might be far more appropriate than any further optical assessment if any major disease is detected at this stage. For a routine examination in the absence of such presenting symptoms, most optometrists will carry out ophthalmoscopy either prior to or after refraction.

Ophthalmoscopy prior to refraction has the advantage of detecting any pathology that might impact upon visual acuity prior to visual assessment. It may also, in rare cases such as early papilledema, reveal important pathology warranting immediate referral and avoiding wasted time in the consulting room. Furthermore, in an ideal world there should be no time constraints upon examination, but this is rarely the case and incorporating ocular examination in the middle of the routine ensures that, if there is not time for all tests to be completed at this visit, at least this major assessment is included. On the other hand, there is the problem of after-images, which may be quite prolonged in the case of certain maculopathies, and which may detract from visual assessment (though retinoscopy is going to introduce another bright target anyway).

Extraocular examination

Very few practitioners have limited access to a slit-lamp nowadays and so the authors would encourage its use on all patients to assess the integrity of the external eye and surrounding structures (Figure 10.1). If not available, or in a domiciliary setting, some information may be gained using a direct ophthalmoscope and many still use a simple hand-held loupe with a pen-torch or hand-held slit-beam torch. If a slit-lamp is not available, then the absolute minimum requirement would be to look for any lesions on the lids, lashes and surrounding skin, the conjunctiva, the cornea

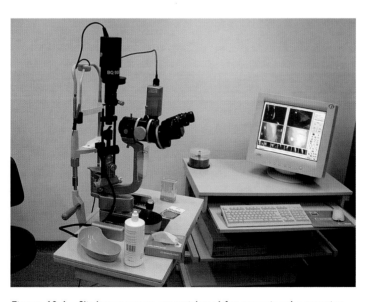

Figure 10.1 Slit-lamps are an essential tool for assessing the anterior eye and adnexa

and the iris. At this stage, anything suspicious should be examined further under the better magnification and the controlled light available on a slit-lamp.

A useful slit-lamp routine is as follows:

- Using diffuse illumination scan the lids, first the lower lid, inferior bulbar and palpebral conjunctiva. Pull the lower lid gently (eversion) to expose the fornix.
- Scan the upper lid and superior bulbar and palpebral conjunctiva. Lid eversion is advisable if there are suspicious signs or symptoms (foreign body sensation, itchiness, redness, etc.) or in any new contact lens candidate.
- Scan temporal bulbar conjunctiva, while patient looking nasally.
- Increase magnification and using an optic section position the beam at the temporal limbus to perform van Herrick angle estimation. You can increase intensity momentarily to allow an easier assessment of the angle.
- Scan the cornea beginning at the temporal side using a 1–2 mm parallelopiped. Switch the beam position to the nasal side and continue scanning the rest of the cornea.
- Use an optic section for nasal van Herick angle estimation at the nasal limbus. This may entail rotating the patient's head on the headrest.
- Continue to scan the nasal bulbar conjunctiva, while patient looking temporally. At this point remember to lower the magnification and use a wider beam.
- Scan temporally again to evaluate the iris. A transillumination technique may be required in order to detect iris atrophies or pigment loss. The anterior chamber can also be assessed at this stage by reducing the height of the beam to a pencil beam, which is expected to be optically empty. Pigment on the endothelium also shows up well against retro-light from the iris or retina.
- Finally, the lens can be examined using a 1 mm parallelepiped or an optic section. First scan the lens by focusing in the anterior capsule, cortex and nucleus. Later focus further into the more posterior layers of the lens. Full visibility of the lens will be restricted by the iris, so a dilated pupil is ideal when a thorough assessment is required.

Intraocular examination

For viewing posterior to the iris, dilation of the pupil is desirable in all cases, though it has to be said that this is rarely common practice, primarily due to time constraints in many busy practices. Until such a time is reached in the UK when the routine eye examination is perceived as both a health check **and** an assessment of refractive error, rather than the onus being on the latter aspect, this situation is likely to continue. However, the authors stand by the sentiment that for all initial examinations, all patients with small pupils or hazy media, symptomatic patients and those in risk categories (such as myopes), should have their pupils be dilated prior to adequate fundus examination. If this is not done, then the burden lies on the practitioner to justify why not.

Probably for historic reasons rather than any others, the direct ophthalmoscope is the preferred means of examining intraocular structures in the UK and still this is supported by UK teaching establishments. This is so despite the fact that the monocular direct view often gives a poor field of view, is difficult through non-transparent media, gives poor contrast of some pigmented lesions, is dependent on refractive error (high myopes, for example, are particularly difficult due to the great magnification of the image) and makes viewing peripheral fundus a haphazard task. Having said this, the use of a direct ophthalmoscope yields best results if the following sequence is adhered to:

- To gain the best field of view, the instrument needs to be very close to the patient's eye. To ensure this is the case and to avoid uncomfortable or embarrassing contact, the practitioner should place their thumb on the patient's brow. This not only serves as a buffer and guide, but also helps to steady the lid when the patient is asked to look downward (Figure 10.2).
- Turning the wheel on the instrument clockwise introduces more positive lenses, anticlockwise more negative. The best view of any particular structure for individual patients and practitioners will vary every time, depending on the refractive error of both patient and practitioner and the distance

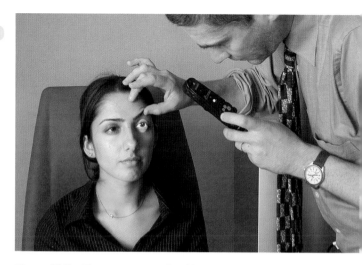

Figure 10.2 The practitioner should place their thumb on the patient's brow, to serve as a buffer and guide, and also help to steady the lid

from the structure being viewed. Good practice therefore involves continually turning the wheel to maximize the clarity of each view. The forefinger held on the wheel at all times facilitates this.

- The practitioner should first view the external eye from a distance of around 5 cm or so. This will usually require a positive lens of several diopters, but turning the wheel while viewing rather than presetting the number will likely allow for a clearer focus. Viewing external structures and then the iris will supplement any major slit-lamp examination (as above) but may in some circumstances be the sole external examination (for example in a domiciliary setting). If this is the case, then great care must be taken to look for disease of the lids and surrounding skin, conjunctiva, cornea and anterior chamber.
- Once focused on the iris, one anticlockwise click of the lenses should put the focus at the plane of the crystalline lens. Most lens opacities will be visible as light-colored areas in this position and movement of the ophthalmoscope may exploit

parallax to establish whether the lesion is anterior to the nodal point of the eye. For the very common cortical changes seen especially in the elderly, the patient should be directed to look in the four major directions of gaze allowing the examiner to look into the superior, temporal, inferior and nasal aspects of the lens and to note (usually with a sketch) any opacification.

- Two or three further anticlockwise clicks of the lens wheel should place the focus into the posterior chamber where it is useful to ask the patient to look upward briefly and then forward again. Waiting for 5 seconds or so after this may allow the practitioner to look for any movement of floaters within the vitreous which, again, should be noted if seen.

- Further anticlockwise clicks should bring the retina into focus and the practitioner should direct their gaze initially to the disk. Except in the case of uncorrected high myopia, the practitioner should be close enough to the patient now to see most of the disk in a single view and their head should now be up against the thumb on the patient's brow (Figure 10.3).

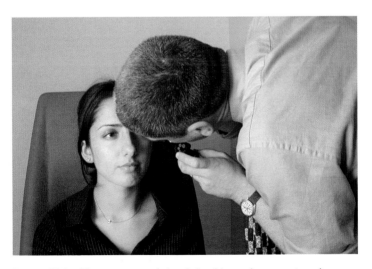

Figure 10.3 The practitioner's head should now be up against the thumb on the patient's brow

- For most undilated pupils the medium-size stop on the instrument should be adequate.
- As a minimum, some note should be made of the distinctness and nature of the disk margin, the vessels at the disc, the color and thickness of the neuroretinal rim (looking to see if it follows the ISNT rule: thickest inferiorly, then superiorly, then nasally and finally temporally) and the vertical CD ratio. Any individual features, such as venous pulsation, vessel bayoneting, peripapillary atrophy and so on, should also be noted. The CD ratio alone is as good as meaningless.
- The practitioner should then scan throughout the posterior pole in a systematic fashion noting particularly the vessels and the background throughout. The same should then be done for more peripheral retina by first asking the patient to look up, up to the left, to the left and so on covering eight positions of gaze in all. This should allow for a reasonable view of most of the fundus, certainly out to the mid-periphery.
- Finally, after changing to the macular stop and ensuring as close a working distance as possible, the practitioner should view the disk and then track the beam temporally until reaching the fovea where a note should be made of the integrity or otherwise of the reflex.
- Where a high myope needs to be viewed, a better field is achieved if the patient is corrected, either by a contact lens or by using a high minus trial lens immediately in front of their eye.

An indirect method, such as the use of a slit-lamp biomicroscopy lens, overcomes most of the disadvantages of the direct instrument suggested above. It is also perfectly possible to adequately view most of the posterior pole without dilation if this is not possible for an acceptable reason. A technique for using a fundus viewing biomicroscopy lens is as follows (adapted from Eperjesi and Ruston in Doshi and Harvey, 2003):

- Position the patient comfortably at the slit-lamp microscope (SLM). Ensure the lens is spotlessly clean and that the magnification is set to low.

- Select a beam height approximately equal to the patient's pupil diameter and a width of about 3 mm.
- Pull the SLM back toward the practitioner and laterally align the slit-beam so that the blurred slit-beam illuminates the center of the patient's pupil.
- Interpose the BIO lens centrally and at about 2 cm from the eye. It is generally not important which way round the BIO lens is held. The surfaces must be clean.
- The SLM should then be moved forward toward the patient and focused on the aerial image of the patient's inverted pupil. Then continue moving forward to focus through the pupil onto the retina. This image is between the BIO lens and the aerial image of the pupil/iris.
- The BIO lens should then be moved forward toward the patient to enlarge the pupil image and, by doing so, increase the field of view (Figure 10.4).
- The practitioner should then scan over the fundus using the same approach adopted when scanning the cornea.

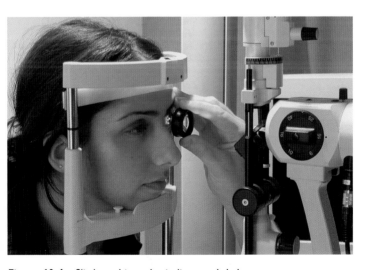

Figure 10.4 Slit-lamp binocular indirect ophthalmoscopy overcomes many of the disadvantages of the direct ophthalmoscope

- The patient should be instructed to look in the different directions of gaze (eight positions) and the lens repositioned each time to optimize the view, tilting where necessary to avoid reflections.
- The magnification can be increased where necessary. The amount of magnification is limited by the particular slit-lamp used.
- Finally, the patient is asked to look toward the practitioner's ear (right ear for right eye, left ear for left eye), which enables visualization of the disc.
- If the vitreous is to be examined, the microscope must be pulled back and the focus shifted onto the floater or hyaloid membrane. Visualization of the vitreous is difficult and the practitioner is recommended to begin with patients who have widely dilated pupils and who have suffered posterior vitreous detachment.
- If necessary the field of view can be increased by moving the lens either vertically or horizontally in the frontal plane. The lens is moved in the same direction to the region that requires investigation. For example, if more of the superior fundus needs to be imaged, then the patient is instructed to look up as far as possible and the lens is moved upward.

It is worth noting that many practitioners fail to achieve a stereoscopic view. This may be confirmed by closing one then the other eye and noting that the fundus view is seen in only one eyepiece. This is invariably due to the viewing lens not being held at the correct working distance from the patient's eye and should be rectified, usually by moving it closer.

11
Prescribing, advice and record-keeping

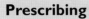
Prescribing

The optometrist is legally bound to issue the patient with a confirmation of their refractive correction, if any, and a note as to the need for any further medical assessment if the eyes were found to be less than healthy. This "prescription" needs to be dated, signed and have details of the prescribing practice and of the patient on it. It is important to remember that the final prescription might be adapted in some way from the final refractive error measurement, for example:

- Where a patient is used to a slightly overminussed correction used primarily for distance viewing and prefers the extra minus.
- Where the refractive error is helping to stabilize binocular state (over-minus to compensate for an exophoria, maximum plus for an accommodative esophoria state).
- Where a reduced post-cycloplegic correction has been decided upon to improve compliance with an isometric hypermetropic refractive error.

The optometrist should also be able to offer advice (and record such on the notes) about the best methods of correction, whether it be contact lenses or a particular spectacle lens form or design. This may aid the subsequent dispensing, particularly if the advice is verbally relayed to the practitioner carrying out any subsequent dispense.

Communication of findings

The delivery of information based upon the findings is the culmination of all the preceding verbal and practical techniques. If the presenting problem of the patient is to be addressed and perhaps resolved, then the recommendations should be delivered in a meaningful way to the patient. To some extent this will depend upon the nature of the underlying problem and the individual patient, and specific examples will be dealt

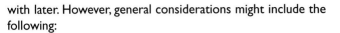

with later. However, general considerations might include the following:

- The recommendation should be clear and concise. After a lengthy summing up and appraisal of the situation it is quite soul-destroying to hear the words "So, do I need glasses then?"
- The recommendation should be specific. "You need to wear your glasses for driving." "You should make an appointment with your GP in the next two days."
- Nonverbal cues help to reinforce the information given, of particular importance if emphasizing an issue with possible health consequences.
- Categorization or presenting information in manageable "chunks" makes information easier to understand and easier to remember, so improving compliance. "You do require new distance glasses. Your current readers are absolutely fine to continue with. Your eyes appear to be healthy. There is no significant change in the health of your eyes since the last examination. I shall want to examine you again in one year." Be very careful not to overload the patient with information as this may decrease subsequent recall of information.
- Where there is a greater amount of detail to be imparted, it is a useful technique to repeat any information of particular importance. Furthermore, if a sequence of information "chunks" is delivered, the patient will tend to remember most the first thing said to them (the primacy effect) and the last thing said to them (the recency effect) and this can be exploited by the skilled practitioner in conveying information.
- The patient should be given ample opportunity to question or respond to any particular points. This will also have the advantage of signifying their understanding of a particular point, so allowing the practitioner to reinforce by repetition or clarification.
- The patient should be made aware of the opportunity for future contact in cases where there may be a problem arising from subsequent consideration of the results.
- Some practitioners give written reinforcement in particular situations where advice may be technical or specific,

for example with regard to a particular lens material or contact lens solution regime.

The conclusion of the examination may often benefit from a call for commitment from the patient, for example, "So I can rely upon you to consult your GP this week?" or "Do you agree that glasses may help to alleviate this problem?"

A note about record-keeping and the Data Protection Act

The Data Protection Act (DPA) came into force in 1998. The law was designed to ensure that information held about any party was secure, available to the party and held in accordance with and in the knowledge of a central agency. Optometrists and opticians hold a good deal of medical information about their patients and customers, much of it in electronic form, and therefore it is important for all eyecare practitioners to be aware of the implications of and their obligations under the law. It is also reasonably common for practitioners to be contacted by unofficial advisors, offering their services for often inflated fees, promising to ensure that the practitioners are operating within the law. Though it is true that any practitioner may easily be operating outside the law if uncertain about their obligations, it is usually a simple matter of familiarizing themselves with these obligations to ensure safe and legal practice and not to give in to some of these opportunistic and clearly out-for-profit fear-mongers.

A brief history

The dramatic increase in the use of computers to hold personal information about people led to the introduction of the Data Protection Act in 1984. This Act offered people the right to have some freedom of access to this information and, where there was proof of exploitation of the information, the right to claim some form of compensation. The law was expanded specifically for health records in 1987 (SI 1987/193 Data Protection

(Subject Access Modification) (Health) Order). This law also saw the establishment of the Data Protection Registrar, to whom a complainant could apply where a breach of the Act was suspected and with whom anyone holding data was required to register.

The Access to Health Records Act 1990 (effective from 1991 to 1998) clarified the process whereby an individual had the right of access to any health record concerning them held by a health professional (including a registered optician) and the right to amend such records where error could be demonstrated. The definition of records in this case excluded any information as described in section 21 of the 1984 DPA.

The Data Protection Act of 1998 superseded the Access to Health Records Act 1990 and in effect combined the two provisions and applies to information stored both electronically and manually. The 1990 Act still applies to deceased patients where information had been stored prior to 1998 who had passed away before this date. As far as patient access to information is concerned, the newer Act allows patients full access to all health records kept about them, and includes access for applicants acting on behalf of the patient, for example in the case of a parent wanting access to information about their child, someone designated in a written statement as having permission to act on behalf of the patient, or when a court has designated someone to act on behalf of a patient otherwise incapacitated and unable to act for themselves. Access may only be refused where it is arguable by the professional that information disclosure may present a danger to the physical or mental state of the applicant.

When the newer DPP effectively repealed the older Access to Health Records Act, there were concerns raised at the time by various civil liberty groups. These included the apparent loss of a patient's right to have a note of their concerns about a disputed matter added to the record, the apparent rise in the fee chargeable by the professional for responding to an application from £10 to a maximum of £50, and the extension of the time allowed for the practitioner to respond to a request from 21 days (where access is required to information recorded within the last 40 days) to a standard 40-day limit under the new DPA. Generally speaking, however, the repeal clarified procedure and, as is often the case in law, is adaptable to changing circumstance. An example of how advice regarding a new demand requires a new clarification is with the new requirements of the proposed pre-registration year where a College of Optometrists assessor requires access to records in order to assess the pre-reg as competent in a certain area. This access will need to be sanctioned by the relevant government body.

The Data Protection Act 1988

The new DPA came into effect on 1 March 2000, and covers all data traceable to an individual held either manually or electronically. An individual has the right to expect the information held about them to be accurate and used only for a specific purpose which needs to be made clear to them (for example, "I am going to make some notes so we can properly monitor how your eyes change over the years"). The right to amend information if inaccurate is maintained and also there is offered the right for an individual to object to the use of data if that use causes harm or distress.

Importantly, practitioners are required to register as data controllers with the Data Protection Registrar, now more commonly known as the Information Commissioner. Failure to register, as well as failure to comply with the provisions outlined, constitutes a criminal offense.

A data controller is defined as "a person who determines the purposes for which, and the manner in which, personal data are, or are to be, processed". This may be an individual practitioner or an organization, such as, for example, a multiple group. A data processor is defined as "a person who processes information on behalf of the data controller", as would be the case of an employee of a multiple or within a registered practice. The patient about whom information is kept is described as the "data subject".

In cases where a data controller is deemed to have failed to satisfy their requirement under the DPA, such as in the case where a practitioner refuses access to a record to a patient, the Information Commissioner may issue an Enforcement Notice.

This sets out the actions the practitioner needs to follow in order to comply with the relevant part of the DPA as well as offering a period within which the practitioner might appeal. Failure to comply may result in court action. The Commissioner may also issue an Information Notice (see below).

Electronic data

As already stated, it is the responsibility of the practitioner (data controller) to notify the Information Commissioner's Office of their activities when they are storing (or "processing") information about a data subject (patient) with some exemptions. Where none of the "processing" is carried out by computer, there is no need to notify. Computer here, however, is a broad enough definition to include image and data storage in instrumentation, audio and CCTV systems. Administrative records (appointments for example), advertising and staff-related information are exempt from the requirement to notify. As most records relate to healthcare, clinical management and possible treatment they are not exempt along with the administrative information. In most cases, therefore, practitioners are bound to notify the Commissioner's Office.

The use of an electronic field screener (even if the results are printed out for storage in the record card) would still require notification, and certainly image storage or topographic data would fall under the DPA requirement. It is surprising how much of a modern optometry practice involves electronic handling of data and therefore notification is the norm.

The electronic optometrist

The patient journey at a modern practice might include the following steps, most of which might be argued as notifiable under the DPA:

- Remote access to a practice website to make an appointment and check information about ocular health and services offered.

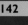
This might be in response to an electronically generated reminder letter.
- CCTV surveillance on entering the practice.
- Personalized computerized information slideshow in waiting area.
- Autorefraction, automated lens meter, tonometry data "hardwired" to a central processor unit.
- Visual fields data stored and compared with previous results.
- Fundus imaging.
- Topography and scanning laser topography or interferometry with analysis of previous and current data compared to stored regression analysis data from trial population.
- Slit-lamp-based external video and image capture.
- PDA-based note-keeping and download of information about patient medication and systemic health condition.
- Automated and variably preprogrammed refraction unit with transfer of result to dispensing unit.
- Video facial measurement and photographic representation of frames on face (and cosmetic contact lenses).
- Electronic data transfer to lab for glazing and to GP for notification of ocular health status.
- Dedicated and personalized information sheets produced for patient to take away.

Even in the case where a data controller is exempt from notification (no electronic processing of clinical data which could influence the clinical management is proven), the practitioner still needs to adhere to the eight principles of the DPA as follows. The data processed must be:

- Fairly and lawfully processed
- Processed for limited purposes
- Adequate, relevant and not excessive
- Accurate
- Kept no longer than necessary (see below)
- Processed in accordance with the data subject's rights
- Secure
- Not transferred without adequate protection

With regard to length of data storage (to comply with the fifth rule above), the UK College of Optometrists specify that data be kept a minimum of 10 years for hospital records, 8 years in general practice, 15 years if the data is involved in clinical trials, and up until the 25th birthday of a child (26th if they were 17 at the conclusion of the treatment or 8 years after the sad event of a child's death).

The Commissioner is also responsible for enforcing the Telecommunications (Data Protection and Privacy) Regulations 1999 and the law that superseded this, the Privacy and Electronic Communications Regulations 2003. These include directions concerning the security of information to be transferred electronically, as well as limitations upon electronic marketing and correspondence, applicable where a practitioner may wish to contact patients through an electronic medium that might be construed as generating "spam". If "teleoptometry" catches on (the paper-free storage and transfer of clinical material) these regulations will become more significant.

Notification is the process by which a data controller's processing details are added to a register. Under the DPA every data controller who is processing personal data needs to notify unless they are exempt. Failure to notify is a criminal offense. Even if a data controller is exempt from notification, they must still comply with the principles.

The Commissioner maintains a public register of data controllers available at www.dpr.gov.uk. A register entry only shows what a data controller has told the Commissioner about the type of data being processed. It does not name the people they hold information about.

Freedom of Information Act 2000

The Freedom of Information Act sits alongside the Data Protection Act 1998 and the forthcoming Environmental Information Regulations as the principal mechanism for access to information held by English, Welsh and Northern Irish public bodies.

The Act does not apply to Scottish public authorities, who fall under the Freedom of Information (Scotland) Act 2002, which is overseen by a separate organization, the Office of the Scottish Information Commissioner. From 1 January 2005 it will oblige opticians' and optometrists' practices to respond to requests about the NHS-related information that it holds, and it will create a right of access to that information.

Summary

Many aspects of modern optometric practice mean that most practitioners act as data controllers to some extent and awareness of their responsibilities under the DPA is essential. Details of notification and responsibilities to the Information Commissioner are available from the Office of the Information Commissioner, Wycliffe House, Water Lane, Wilmslow, Cheshire, SK9 5AF (tel. 01625 545740). Do this yourself and avoid paying extortionate amounts for less than respectable outfits offering their services to do so at an exorbitant fee.

Useful references

http://www.hmso.gov.uk/acts/acts1990
http://www.hmso.gov.uk/acts/acts1998
http://www.hmso.gov.uk/acts/acts2000
http://www.informationcommissioner.gov.org

References

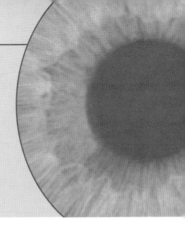

Barrat CD (1945) Sources of error and working methods in retinoscopy.
    Brit. J. Physiol. Opt. **5**:35–40

Bennett AG, Francis JL (1962) Ametropia and its correction. In *The Eye* ed.
    Davison H, Vol. IV, pp. 131–80. Academic Press, New York

Doshi S, Harvey W (2003) *Investigative Techniques and Ocular Examination*, chap. 9,
    Assessment of the fundus (Eperjesi F & Ruston D). Butterworth-Heinemann,
    Oxford

Elliott DB (2003) *Clinical Procedures in Primary Eye Care,* chap. 1, p. 9. Butterworth-
    Heinemann, Oxford

Ettinger ER (1994) *Professional Communication in Eye Care,* chap. 3, p. 44.
    Butterworth-Heinemann, Oxford

Evans BJW (1997) *Pickwell's Binocular Vision Anomalies*, 3rd ed., pp. 65–6.
    Butterworth-Heinemann, Oxford

Francis JL (1973) The axis of a astigmatism with special reference to streak
    retinoscopy. *Brit. J. Physiol. Op.,* **12**:11–22

Humphriss D (1984) *Refraction Science and Psychology.* Juta & Co., Cape Town

Jennings JAM, Charman WN (1973) A comparison of errors in some methods of
    subjective refraction. *Ophthal. Opt.* **13**:8

Mallett RFJ (1964) The investigation of heterophoria at near and a new fixation
    disparity technique. *Optician* **148**:573–81

Mallett RFJ (1988) Techniques of investigation of binocular vision anomalies.
    In *Optometry* (ed. Edwards KH & Llewellyn RD), pp. 238–69. Butterworth-
    Heinemann, Oxford

Manny R, Hussein M, Scheimann M, Kurz D, Neimann K, Zinzer K and the Comat
    Study Group (2001) Tropicamide 1%: An effective cycloplegic agent for myopic
    children. *Invest. Ophthalmol. Vis. Sci.* **42**:1728–35

McBrien N, Taylor SP (1986) Effect of fixation target on objective refraction. *Am. J.
    Optom. Physiol. Opt.* **63**:346–50

Millodot M, Millodot S (1989) Presbyopia correction and the accommodation in
    reserve. *Ophthal. Physiol. Opt.* **9**:126–32

Mohindra I (1975) A technique for infant visual examination. *Am. J. Optom.*
    52:867–70

References

North R, Henson DB (1981) Adaption to prism induced heterophoria in subjects with abnormal binocular vision or asthenopia. *Am. J. Optom. Physiol. Opti.* **58(A)**:746–52

O'Leary D (1988) Subjective refraction. In *Optometry* (ed. Edwards KH & Llewellyn RD), p. 126. Butterworth-Heinemann, Oxford

Parker JA (1996) Stationary streak retinoscopy. *Can. J. Ophthalmol.* **1**:228–239

Safir A, Hyams L, Philpott J. (1970) Studies in refraction. I. The precision of retinoscopy. *Arch. Ophthalmol.* **84**:49–61

Saunders K, Westall C (1992) Comparison between near retinoscopy and cycloplegic retinoscopy in the refraction of infants and children. *Optomo. Vis. Sci.* **69**:615–22

Taylor S (1988) Retinoscopy. In *Optometry* (ed. Edwards KM & Llewellyn RD), p. 85. Butterworth-Heinemann, Oxford

Viner C (2004) Refractive examination. In Harvey W, Gilmartin B, *Paediatric Optometry*, p. 24. Butterworth-Heinemann, Oxford

Westheimer G (1959) Accommodation levels during near crossed cylinder test. *Am. J. Optom.* **35**:599–604

Index

Index